Contents

D0496001

Introducing our main models. From left, Alex, Joyce, Sally and the author, Ian.

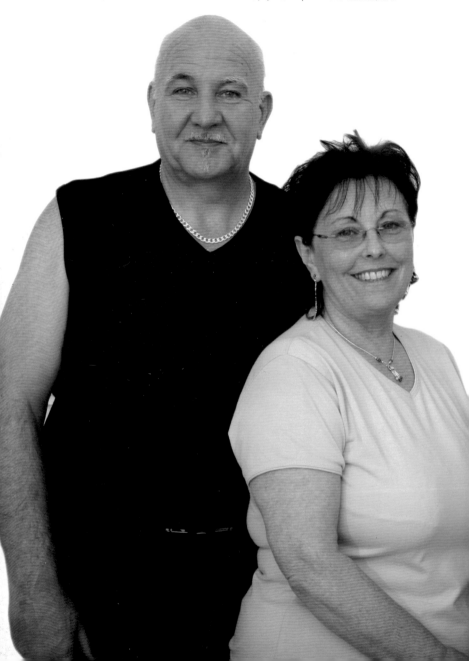

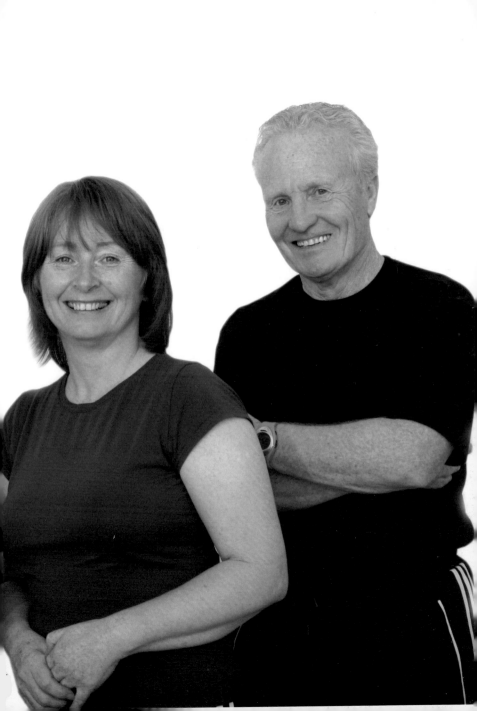

Foreword

The purpose of this book was simply to persuade people over 50 (and those approaching 50) that fitness and health can be attained or improved by physical activity at any age. For this reason I have set out to offer suggestions on various forms of exercise for people ranging from the (presently) totally unfit to those who are already very fit but who would welcome the invigoration that comes from trying new or challenging activities.

I have deliberately limited the use of scientific, anatomical or medical information; it has been my experience that my target audience will ignore information regarding actin and myosin, mitochondria and Golgi apparatus, cut to the chase instead, and get on with it. It is, alternatively, possible that readers may use this book to jam the door open while taking the empties to the dustbin. The choice, of course, is yours, and I hope you will get involved, for your own sake. Good luck, whichever you decide.

Ian Oliver

Acknowledgements

I am deeply indebted to many people for their assistance in putting this book together. Some of us share a common view that the over 50's have spent too long in the exclusion zone where exercise is concerned, and that so much more can be done to get people involved in prolonging their lives while adding to the quality of it. If a dozen or more older folk get into training and actually discover they enjoy it, then writing this book has been worthwhile.

Thanks are especially extended to:

- Savash Mustafa (Osteopath), my medical guru
- Victoria Mose (Course Tutor, Y.M.C.A Fitness Industry Training) my fitness second opinion
- Rob Springett, swimming supremo
- Mike Smith and Mike Jackson, my cycling experts
- Samantha Russell, my bands and tubes buff
- Johnny 'Father' Wahlers, my tennis 'ace'
- Terry Barnett and Steve Wright, of the 'tough guys do Pilates' school.
- Joyce Mose, Sally Bladon, Doug Mather and "Big Al" Livingstone, my brave yet mainly willing 'guinea pigs'.
- Colleagues: Cheryl Power, Wayne Rowlands and Owen Ogbourne for their support, encouragement and opinions (or abuse) throughout - just wait until they're 50.
- Bob and Judy Breen of the Bob Breen Academy for letting me use the gym as if I owned it – cheers.
- Sandra Heeney and Ann Taylor, the Academy's golden girls
- Harry and Tricia Newson for letting me take their names in vain.
- Boundless gratitude to Emma, Gilly, Anna and James at Snowbooks – such patience.

Dedication

Dedicated to all instructors, staff and students (especially my Monday Mobs) of the Bob Breen Academy past and present – even the ones still under 50.

To Brenda, Marge, Sue, Jimmy, Tom, Glen, Jane, Ellie, Joe, Charmaine, Clare, Danny and Ronnie, and all the Walkers and Mitchells.

To the memory of John McDavid, Laura Logan, Andrew "Wink" Walker, Roy Beckworth, Johnny Bird, Mag and Archie, F.S.O and that all-swimming all-dancing gal, Dolly Walker – dance on, Doll.

"Physical fitness is the first requisite of happiness. In order to achieve happiness, it is imperative to gain mastery of your body. If at the age of 30 you are stiff and out of shape, you are old. If at 60 you are supple and strong then you are young."

Joseph Hubertus Pilates

1. Before You Start - Medical Clearance

If you have any concerns about your health then I must stress the importance of getting clearance from your doctor before starting physical activity. This would be advisable, especially if you have never participated in physical exercise before, or not since your youth. Be prepared to start gradually and take the easier options when you first start. Exercise does not have to hurt or be excessively strenuous to be effective. You should, and my fervent hope is that you will, enjoy exercising.

My favourite quote on the subject comes from Dr. Per-Olaf Astrand of Sweden who declared:

> "There is less risk in activity than in continuous inactivity... It is more advisable to pass a careful medical examination if you intend to be sedentary."

> (Astrand & Rodahl, 1970)

> *"Old age will only be respected if it fights for itself, maintains its rights, avoids dependence on anyone and asserts control over its own to its last breath"*
>
> Marcus Tullius Cicero (106 - 43 BC)

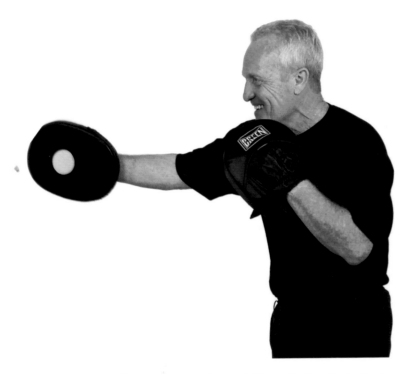

The author, Ian Oliver, training on focus pads at the Bob breen Academy, Hoxton, London

2. Becoming a Rock of Ages

I feel I should point out that I am not a doctor, physiologist or kinesiologist and that my only qualifications are as a fitness instructor, which I have been longer than I care to remember.

Although I have no medical training, my good friend and former colleague, the redoubtable osteopath Savash Mustafa, has checked out my recommendations to ensure they are not life-threatening; especially as my main intention is to prolong a healthy life. I have also benefited from the invaluable assistance of my colleague Victoria Mose, a Senior Instructor at the YMCA Training and Development Department, and a veritable font of fitness knowledge.

I have deliberately not included details of how muscles, blood and nerve systems work, as:

1. There are more specifically scientific books that will describe this in detail

2. It has been my experience that, upon opening a fitness book, people will skim through, or most likely skip altogether, the 'science bit', so that they can just get on with it. (I must admit to doing it myself.)

My advice is drawn from my personal experience of trying to get people (of all ages, shapes, sizes, and fitness levels) fit or fitter. I must place emphasis on the word 'trying' as I have not been without my failures; many people start out keen but do not have what I call 'stick-ability', the will to hang on when the workload becomes challenging.

I should also point out that I am not a thirty-something who knows exercise theory and practice inside out but doesn't know how a 63 year old man will feel once he tries it; I am the 63 year old man. So, not only am I qualified to say how it feels, I have already have done 99% of it, at one time or another, and a great deal of it recently.

At the age of fifty-plus you have come to a fork in the road; one direction leads to inactivity and a slow decline in health and movement, and the other (far less travelled) leads to exercise and positive health improvement.

So ask yourself if you really feel you have stick-ability; there is only one way to find out, and I wish you luck in your journey.

> "Add life to years not just years to life'
>
> Motto of The American Gerontological Society.

3. What Kind of Training?

Much of the training I advocate in this book is the way I still train. I admit to be something of a training nut – when only three or four people turned up for training on a foul night in sheeting rain, I would be one of them. I still enjoy running, weight training, swimming (when I get the chance), boxing training, core training and my latest love, golf, which I used to loathe. I was dragged kicking and screaming to golf by my wife, who often returns a better score than me, but had to admit it provides not just good gentle exercise in a healthy environment, but a test of one's patience and spirit. It makes me wish I'd started 40 years ago but unfortunately where I was raised in East London there was a distinct lack of golfing opportunities. The point I make here is that you are never too old to try it out. You may, like me, become a convert to something you had previously missed out on.

I have friends of around my own age who are as fit, or fitter than myself; the 'use it or lose it' principle applies here, especially with strength and flexibility. If we want to maintain our strength, suppleness, vitality and, essentially, our "marbles" as we grow older we have to run (not literally!) to stay in place.

As we grow older a gradual strength loss will occur, but resistance training, especially with weights, can still bring gains. Tests have shown the over-80's can still make impressive strength gains and even change muscle size. One piece of research states "muscle responds to vigorous training with marked and rapid improvement into the ninth decade of life" (Fiatarone Singh M. A et al., 2000). How impressive is that – building muscle strength in your nineties? Strength improvements through resistance training depend, as with younger people, on the frequency, duration and intensity applied by the individual.

A good quality magazine for older trainers, *Masters Athletics Monthly,* gives staggering details of record-breaking feats by runners in their 70's, 80's and even 90's. In October 2004 Scotland's Gordon Porteous is reported to have recorded the fastest time for the over-90's at 10,000 metres (69:26.92) But then he has been competing since 1935, thus showing the value of continuous exercise. It was a stunning achievement, but he did however admit "my knees were knackered" – really, no kidding! (Detail from *Masters Athletics Monthly,* issue 3, December 2004).

Anybody who has seen ex-Mr Universe Bill Pearl at the age of 75, with a physique 20 and 30-something bodybuilders would kill a close relative to attain, can see that the potential does not just fade away where strength training is concerned.

Consider also the staggering "*7 marathons in 7 days*" achievement of Sir Ranulph Fiennes (regardless of his other outstanding feats of super-human endurance) despite having undergone heart surgery, a double bypass no less, only 4 months earlier.

I am not going to advocate, as I have seen in fitness books for the mature person, that a little regular gardening, taking the stairs instead of the lift, vacuuming, or even occasional dancing (excellent exercise that it is) will suffice. I am trying to instill a commitment to regular, structured training, in which I hope you will find enough interest, inspiration and feelings of self-worth and well-being to give you the stick-ability such training requires and deserves.

"Every human being is the author of his own health"

Prince Guatama Sridhar (founder of Buddhism)

4. Introduction

Fifty years ago, at the age of twelve, I was living with my grandparents in Hackney. My grandfather's only form of exercise was to amble approximately a quarter of a mile to the Duke of Richmond pub, at least once a day, occasionally twice. He was around 60 years old, smoked hand-rolled cigarettes, made from Old Holborn tobacco, drank Mackeson stout, showered his food with salt, dumped two teaspoons of sugar into the copious amount of tea he consumed, and was at least two stone overweight. He passed away ten years later from a heart condition. He was, and still is, in my eyes, a wonderful man, and I never gave a thought to the fact he could have stopped smoking, cut down on alcohol and taken more exercise; he had served, in one form or another, in two World Wars and most probably felt he was due some recreation, particularly as most of his peers shared a similar lifestyle. The thought of him jogging around the streets of Hackney in a singlet and shorts is nothing short of hilarious; he still possessed the brown plimsolls the army had issued him with in the First World War – the only athletic apparel he ever possessed. He wore them, minus the laces, in lieu of carpet slippers. He had frequent bouts of illness, which I can now understand, given his lifestyle. In striking contrast my grandmother, two years his senior, was a constant whirl of activity, walking for miles almost daily, gardening at every opportunity, swimming when she could, carrying home heavy bags of shopping on foot rather than wait for buses. The crazy paving in the garden was from large slabs she transported home on my sister's old push-chair, and which she and I laid, while my grandfather perused the racing form in his deckchair. As a result, although asthmatic, she was as tough as nails, and lived to the age of 95, generally enjoying good health.

Exercise, and the benefits to be derived from exercise, were a world away from them, as they were to the great majority of ordinary people in those days.

Teenagers in those days, in my experience, usually detested exercise in the joyless and insipid form it was forced upon us: press-ups, sit-ups, climbing ropes and jumping over wooden benches, beams and pommel horses once a week, at the barking directions of a 'gym-teacher', was not what most youngsters found any stimulation or satisfaction in. In actual fact, so arduous and tedious was the physical activity as organised by educational facilities that most youngsters resolved to give it a wide berth once they had left school, especially the girls. Boys generally continued to enjoy some form of exercise, usually by playing football, cricket, boxing or by taking advantage of the affordable entrance fees of public swimming baths; if you were spartan enough to brave the water at the local open-air pool before 9 o'clock, admittance was free. The thought of playing golf, tennis or skiing was as remote as space travel. Boys' clubs encouraged sporting activity, but there seemed no equivalent for girls, and I don't recall anybody ever questioning it. Go to any gym today, though, and observe the ratio of women to men, and the quantum leap that has occurred regarding women and exercise.

When physical exercise, particularly 'aerobics' and jogging, became all the rage, circa the seventies, a sea-change in public attitude to exercise took place, and the benefits of regular workouts became evident to everybody; whether they would share it or scorn it was another matter.

Gyms sprang up nationwide, sport apparel became fashionable and previously prohibitively expensive sports like golf, tennis, squash and skiing became accessible to working-class folk. Local councils made gyms affordable. To a great extent people became exercise-conscious.

The sad fact is that even today so many of the older generation view exercise as a chore, a cheerless trial to be endured if they want to attain any degree of fitness, while memories of press-ups and long runs being forms of punishment continue to enforce this attitude. The hardest people, in my experience, to get involved in training are the ones who have found their way to the gym by a doctor's referral, or a concerned spouse; many of this reluctant group surprise themselves in the satisfaction they derive from exercise, once they overcome their initial aversion.

The whole point of this book is to combat this image of exercise as a cheerless ordeal; it really can be a lot of fun, as many older people have discovered. Trying a sport or regime you may have never previously considered can bring a freshness you may have never hitherto have envisaged. Most of these activities do not require you to sign up long term; many are organised to allow you to try a 'taster' session. For people who would prefer to strive for improved fitness at home I have attempted to supply alternative, usually more affordable, methods of training.

Age has become less of a barrier to those who are determined or enthusiastic enough to give it their best shot. One vital point to remember is that exercise does not have to hurt to be effective; the 'no pain – no gain' maxim is not the one for you, your motto must become 'use it, or lose it', if you want to get fit, and stay fit. There has never been a better time for mature people to get involved in exercise and sport; there is an abundance of information, an absence of stigma (of the old people training? Whatever next? variety). Hopefully much of the government health directives will take a more active form than mere vocal encouragement, making sport and exercise more freely available and affordable to all.

By 2020 more than half of all British adults will be over 50. Sohan Singh, a former representative of Kenya in the Mr. Universe competition, and a Karate 3rd Dan, who obtained a Master's degree from the Open University in 2004, and works out daily, objected to having to retire from his much-loved job in the probation service, as he had reached 65. As somebody who had sat on the Racial Equality Council for 14 years his comments are significant. He states:

"Ageism is worse than racism or sexism, because there is so little recognition that it is wrong. There is no commission fighting for your rights… ageing is a little bit like disability, in that a lot of the problems are socially created. People may have slightly more or different needs as they get older, but the key thing is to

keep people as human beings, functioning as fully as possible. It is society that imposes on you a sense that you are old. I feel pretty young."

I would like to think that Mr. Singh speaks for many people of his generation, who have been made to feel, by society, worthless or redundant.

Nobody should write themselves off as unsuitable for anything they wish to achieve physically merely because they are 'too old' or 'too out of shape' – there is something for everybody to get involved in. My ardent hope is that this book will help you find it.

Ian Oliver, 1st November 2006

"Fifty is the new thirty"

Andrew Goodsell (SAGA chief executive)

5. Why Exercise?

In our later years physical activity can maintain and improve these essentials:

1. Stamina

_____

2. Muscular strength

_____

3. Flexibility and suppleness

_____

4. Balance and co-ordination

_____

1. Stamina

Stamina is another way of expressing 'staying power', the power of endurance. Whether you are swimming, jogging or just walking briskly your heart is going to be beating faster and your lungs are being exercised, building cardiovascular endurance. As you work faster or for a longer time you will be improving your stamina. Don't attempt to continually extend both distance and duration; wait until one or the other are no longer challenging. Muscular stamina will be improved by lighter weights and higher repetitions (see Weight Training page 206).

2. Muscular strength

Training at any age can improve your strength. Weights spring to mind as the most effective form of resistance training, but body weight exercises and those performed against gravity (covered in calisthenics) are useful if no weights are available.

Stronger muscles make everyday tasks easier, as well as strengthening your joints and back.

3. Flexibility & suppleness

Inactivity over the years will diminish our level of flexibility, it follows the 'use it or lose it' principle. As with strength, a reasonable level of flexibility can help with day to day tasks as well as assisting physical activity. Into the later years it can help with balance and relieving aches and strains (see Flexibility, page 48).

4. Balance and co-ordination

Being confident in maintaining our equilibrium may not seem too important at 50 – we more or less take it for granted. However, in twenty or thirty years time it becomes crucial, often a matter of life and death, given the high number of fatalities, and eventual fatalities, following falls.

Sport helps enormously with co-ordination; in racquet sports, for example, the upper and lower body must co-ordinate. The best training tool for co-ordination is, in my experience, skipping, which is also a good test of balance. Most sports call for some level of specific co-ordination. By trying them or continuing to train in them you can keep improving your ability in this area (see Skipping, page 160). The chart below shows which activities assist primarily with the above:

Activity	Stamina	Strength	Flexibility	Balance	Co-ordination
Swimming	*	*	*		
Dancing			*	*	*
Cycling	*	*		*	
Skipping	*			*	*
Tennis		*			*

Main factors of ill-health and disability in mature years

1. Smoking

2. Excessive body fat

3. Reduced physical activity

I'm quite sure everybody is aware of the risks of the first two but possibly less mindful of the third factor.

The first is a matter of personal choice. We are all aware of the obvious perils of smoking, and I do not intend to preach about something so blatantly obvious.

Regarding excessive body fat, the answer lies not only in exercise but some honest and probably painful examination and adjustment to diet. I would advise you to read up on nutrition and dietary advice from a specialist source, such as Anita Bean's "Sports Nutrition" (2006).

Inadequate physical activity is considered, in the USA, to cause nearly 30% of all deaths from heart disease, colon cancer and diabetes (Martinez Me. 1999). While, in the UK, improved heart disease treatment has brought about declining rates of fatalities, total avoidance of heart and other life-threatening diseases would naturally appear the preferred option; making the change to a more physically active lifestyle can make a huge improvement to your heart, lungs and muscular functions at any age.

So, if you decide you want to live longer, stay strong or get stronger – face the fact that if you're going to be around longer you want to enjoy good health in that time.

> "Physical fitness is not only one of the most important keys to a healthy body, it is the basis of dynamic and creative intellectual activity"
>
> John Fitzgerald Kennedy

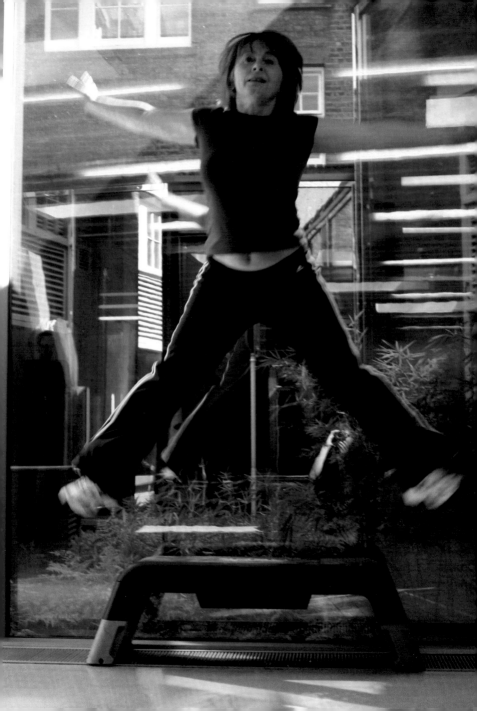

6. Our Health and the Department of Health

"The evidence of the potential health gains from active lifestyles is clear. We need a culture shift to achieve these goals…current levels of physical activity are a reflection of personal attitudes about time use and of cultural and societal values. They also reflect how conducive our homes, neighbourhoods and environment have become for inactive living…if people of all ages can be engaged in a new way of thinking about active lifestyles, better health can be a realistic goal for all. Physical activity needs to be seen as an opportunity – for enjoyment, for improved vitality, for a sense of achievement, for fitness, for optimal weight, and – not least – for health. It needs to be seen as enjoyable, and as fun – not an unnecessary effort. Perceptions also need to be changed – too many people think they are already active enough."

Extract from "At Least Five A Week" by Professor Sir Liam Donaldson, Chief Medical Officer, Department of Health (29th April 2004).

This was taken from, as stated, the chief medical officer's report, which set out to show that at least 30 minutes a day of moderate exercise on five (or more) days a week reduces the risk of premature death from cardiovascular disease and some cancers, as well as the onset of type 2 diabetes. One of the major points raised concerns "time use". One of the main issues people raise in explaining why they cannot exercise is the lack of time, but personal time management is a crucial factor in getting some physical activity done, and thereby prolonging not only the amount of time you will live, but the quality of life you will enjoy by doing so. Often we need to change not only our lifestyle – not always drastically – but our mindset. The report went on to give examples of how the thirty minutes could be composed of bouts of 10 or more minutes of activity throughout the day, not necessarily of strenuous organised exercise, but such activities as mowing the lawn, vacuum cleaning or gardening. The drawback here is that unless you are digging, vigorously clipping a hedge (with shears), or heaving materials to and fro, gardening is usually something of a leisurely affair, a light labour of love, and not usually too labour-intensive for somebody of reasonable health.

Such is the efficiency of the modern appliances we now tend to use: electric mowers and vacuum cleaners reduce most of the effort involved. The sad news is that effective exercise should produce at least a light perspiration, and the feeling that you have exerted yourself.

Compare the amount of calories expended in the following activities; they will vary with individuals dependent on your size and how much effort you apply!

Activity	Calories per minute.
Driving car	2.8
Driving motor bike	3.4
Painting	3.5
Vacuuming	3.5
Sweeping floors	3.9
Ironing	4.2
Gardening (weeding)	5.6

Activity	Calories per minute.
Gardening (digging)	8.6
Cycling (easy)	5.0
Cycling (hard)	15
Dancing (leisurely)	5
Golf	5
Dancing (vigorously)	7.5
Walking (3.5 Mph)	6
Jogging (5 mph)	10
Running (7.5 Mph)	15
Running (10 mph)	20
Swimming (breast stroke/backstroke)	6-12
Swimming (butterfly)	14
Skipping (leisurely)	10
Skipping (fast)	15
Rowing (leisurely)	5
Rowing (strenuously)	15
Badminton (recreational)	5
Badminton (competitive)	10
Table tennis (recreational)	5
Table tennis (competitive)	7.5
Lawn tennis (recreational)	7
Lawn tennis (competitive)	11

Too often we worry about the perception of others; that they will think we are odd or eccentric by participating in activities, particularly once we pass 50. The best procedure in this case is to carry on regardless, and:

- Take the stairs when "normal" people are getting the lift.

- Walk to destinations a mile or two away, allowing time and refusing offered 'lifts' from well-intended friends.

- Go for a swim or exercise class in your lunch break instead of launching into pub or canteen food. Eat something light and sit down for a proper meal at home in the evening. Stay away from the pub unless it's a special social occasion.

- Unless the roads are particularly hazardous, try cycling to and from work. Don't worry about looking silly in a cycling helmet: they are crucial on today's roads.

> "We are happier in many ways when we are old than when we were young. The young sow wild oats, the old grow sage."
>
> Winston Churchill

7. Suggestions for Ageing Well

1. Watch what you eat.

Steer clear of 'quick-fix' diets. Try to stay low in fat in what you eat if you want to stay low in fat in your figure. Drink plenty of water and get your daily ration of fruit and vegetables, ideally five a day.

2. Take regular exercise.

You need to increase your heart rate, ideally with moderate physical activity for 30 minutes 5 times a week – failing this, as often as you can. Don't make excuses in order to avoid it; set the specific time aside.

3. Reduce stress levels.

Take stock of your life; does the choice come down to health versus wealth? Are you still knocking yourself out in your later life to earn as much as possible, regardless of your well-being? Do friends and family hint you might do well to ease off a little? Could you settle for fewer possessions and a better quality of life if that was the choice? When problems arise don't bottle them up – talk to those close to you about them. Take a long walk to think your problems over, leaving your mobile phone at home. Look into meditation; more and more people gain great comfort from it. Buy a book on relaxation techniques.

4. Reduce sunbathing.

Unless you want a face that resembles a saddlebag with eyes, and more worryingly, run the risk of skin cancer, moderate your sunbathing hours and discover the right factor suncream for your type of skin. Check the weather before leaving home if you intend to be out all day – do you need a hat or sunscreen? Given the vagaries of British weather it may be pouring with rain when you leave home but change to blistering sunshine in a short time.

5. Get enough rest.

Don't drink coffee or alcohol before turning in if you can avoid it. Don't go to bed directly after a heavy meal or strenuous exercise. Try 'napping' during the day if you are at home and feel weary; if you can't get off to sleep at night get up and sit in a chair and read, or watch some soporifically mind-numbing late-night television for half an hour.

6. Use your loaf.

Reading the paper, attempting the crossword or Sudoku, learning new skills, possibly at local adult institutes, such as learning a language or gaining computer familiarity, a hobby or therapy – any of these can help to keep you 'switched on'.

Sports and pastimes like darts, snooker, chess and card games may not expend a great deal of energy, but all help enormously to focus the mind.

7. Keep your friends.

If you have good friends, stay in touch with them; one of the benefits of getting older is the number of long-term friendships you have forged. Human contact and communication are essential to keep your sanity and well-being, and give you the chance to share your problems with somebody, whether they want to hear them or not.

> *"At twenty I tried to vex my elders, past sixty it's the young I hope to bother"*
>
> W.H. Auden "Shorts I" 1969

8. Body Types – Know Your Type

We all look the way we do thanks to our genetic make-up and our hormones. Diet and physical activity play an obvious role in our appearance, but do not, as you may have noticed with some bitterness, affect everybody the same way.

As a youngster I worked with a guy named Pete Eddowes, who could eat two dinners to my one in the café. He had energy to burn, was forever hungry and never added an ounce of weight to his long lean frame. What we didn't realise, and he certainly didn't at the time, was that he was an 'ectomorph' – one of three main body types, categorised as 'soma' types.

People can be categorised into three basic 'body types', although this is a very broad generalisation as the three types all usually have the characteristics of one of the other groups – so many of us are something in between. However, the three main types are below.

Ectomorph

Ectomorphs are usually lean, tall types, with narrow shoulders and hips. They are the weight-training instructor's nightmare. Trying to pack muscle on to guys with this frame is a real challenge, as they have a high metabolism and may be able to eat large amounts of food without gaining weight

Mesomorph

Mesomorphs usually have a densely muscled body, with a medium-to-large frame with broad shoulders and narrow hips, medium-to-high metabolism, and are capable of putting on muscle without too much trouble, or fat if they are inactive or overfed.

Endomorph

Endomorphs are unfortunate enough to be endowed with higher body fat levels than they would like, and often have a problem shifting fat, as they usually have a low metabolism. They invariably have a limited amount of muscle mass and size, which usually endows them with a 'pear' shape (wider at the hips).

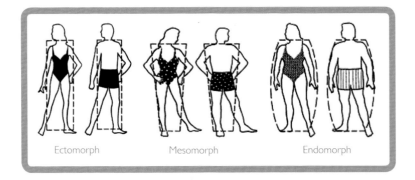

Ectomorph   Mesomorph   Endomorph

As stated it is not as clear-cut as all that. Most people have characteristics from all groups in differing proportions.

The three basic groups became widely referenced in literature about diet, bodybuilding and general exercise, so at least some of the school sports coaches should have had some idea why some children were shaped the way they were and could not help their ample proportions. I always felt sorry for the overweight kids in gym classes; we had a PE master who regarded them on the same footing as war criminals, unaware of the fact they were endomorphs doing their level best.

Conclusion

Although, to an extent, you have to accept your shape, all is not lost; diet and exercise can make large, if not dramatic changes to your body regardless of somatotype, so you can still shape your own destiny. The soma types are only a guide, but they nevertheless help us to be realistic about our ambitions, with regard to our figure.

9. The Double Curse of being Overweight

It's a sad fact that excessive amounts of body fat tend to limit or restrict the ability of the individual to perform physical activity. This results in a decline of overall fitness, which in turn is likely to cause a further accumulation of even more body fat.

Q) How do we break out of this vicious circle?

A) We do something within our own individual capability.

Can an individual be fat and fit? The overweight guys I played football with were usually as fit as the skinny guys, and usually stronger – you wouldn't have wanted a tackle off one of them. Consider the pre-Tyson and Lennox Lewis era heavyweight boxers, invariably carrying a 'spare tyre' around the middle, but capable of incredible levels of fitness and the portly figures (both men and women) swathed in grease that swam the English Channel, often appearing to carry their own built-in lifebelt.

So, do not allow the fact that you are overweight, even heavily overweight, to deter you from getting involved in exercise.

It is better to be fat and active than thin and sedentary!

A moderate, achievable and consistent level of energy output will be a good start. If you are unsure of how much effort you can make, use the 'beginner' levels throughout this book. Aim low to start with; setting yourself hard targets may prove discouraging, start with the easier stuff and take pride in the fact that you are taking a positive step towards fitness.

> If you are overweight and have not done any physical activity for some time – use exercises as advised for LEVEL I (see page 45)

> If you are overweight but active, and have done some physical activity in the recent past – use exercises as advised for LEVEL 2 (see page 45)

Muscles have memories

This is not the title of a sci-fi short story but a matter of fact, if not put in exactly scientific terms. The truth is that people who were active in their younger days (and especially if they have remained moderately active) will have physical capabilities that will far exceed those who have led a sedentary existence. The 'returning factor' means you should not take too long to get back on track; all you need to do is to take it easy when you first start exercising again.

But what if my muscles have no memories?

There is potentially bad news for this group when their doctor informs them 'what you need is some exercise'. The best course is to get involved in some gentle exercise to start with. Do not begin with something that will be excessively punishing, demanding or boring. Keep away from activities that could prove hazardous to your health, such as playing squash (a game for which you have to be fit to start with); there is plenty of time for more vigorous pursuits once you get in appropriate condition. Walking and swimming would be beneficial start-up exercises as neither of these activities place undue stress on the heart or the joints.

Look to take part in something you enjoy doing; getting involved in exercise should not feel like you are doing community service for wrongdoing.

10. Training Levels

Training Levels for the Over-50's.

Identify your level and then once the exercises become easy move up to the next level.

Level 1: the beginner

Total newcomer to physical activity or heavily overweight. Progress to level 2 when you can either walk briskly for 20 minutes in comfort (check on RPE scale page 40) or you feel much fitter in daily tasks (e.g. going upstairs, carrying shopping).

Level 2: the reasonably fit and healthy but unused to regular physical exercise

If you are not sure whether you fit into this category use the RPE scale to check how you feel after 20 minutes of BRISK walking (not ambling – step it up!). Be brutally honest with yourself; if you are unsure, as with any exercise or physical activity, err on the side of caution, and downgrade to beginner.

Level 3: the fit

If you've always been fit, either by dint of having an active occupation, or training moderately, train at this level. If you are at this level, for example, you are capable of jogging in comfort but can't run for more than 30 minutes, or you can plod on the stationary bike but couldn't endure any form of anaerobic exercise for too long.

Level 4: the very fit

Regular exercisers in running, swimming, weight training or comparable pursuits. You can run long distances, row for over 30 minutes on the machine, or swim over half a mile in the comfort zone. You have been training regularly for a long time, possibly since your youth.

I have used the examples above as a very rough guide. I know incredibly fit people who cannot run any distance at all due to chronic back or knee problems, but can swim for miles and row for an hour with no problem at all. Take the self-test on a regular basis, i.e. once a month maximum. Any more can be misleading or depressing. The longer you space these tests out while you are training the more likely you are to be satisfied with your progress. As we age we must expect limitations of movement and suppleness; we cannot, sadly, turn back the clock to how we used to train twenty-five or so years ago, so the need now is to at least preserve, and hopefully improve, what fitness we already have.

F.I.T.

The progress and improvement you make in the course of your exercise will be dependent on three factors, usually described in fitness jargon as F.I.T.

F = frequency (how often you train)

I = intensity (how much effort you make)

T = time spent, the duration of your workout

Don't work too hard at first. Your overload and adaptation should be graduated in small increments.

Don't get frustrated if you move up one level fairly quickly and then plateau on the next level – be patient.

If you are at all unsure of which level you need to be working at, always opt for the LOWER level. There is always scope to then progress safely.

Learn to Rest

To make positive progress in your fitness you have to bear in mind that where exercise is concerned it is often the case that the overused phrase 'less is more' is applicable. Working out non-stop (even if you had the capacity to) without rest would be foolhardy. While you are training muscle-fibre is broken down (this is known as micro trauma). Essential repairs to strengthen muscles take place while you rest them. For this reason, and to prevent unnecessary soreness, weight training requires a day or two between sessions, unless you are at an extremely advanced or experienced stage of development.

If you don't feel well – DON'T TRAIN, JUST REST.

A short lay-off will not bring about a decline in your progress, but you will be advised to take it easy for the initial sessions when you return to activity.

Make sure you get adequate sleep; sleep deprivation can hamper your performance levels. Hopefully your earlier exertion will help the advancement of getting off to sleep shortly after your head hits the pillow. If you feel the need during the day, take a short 'power nap' when you get the chance (look on it as battery-charging) – preferably at home as this may attract attention at the gym.

Take it Lying Down

A simple technique, taken from the teachings of the Alexander Technique, referred to as the 'semi-supine position', can prove extremely beneficial. Simply lie on a carpeted floor, or an exercise mat, with your head resting on a book (the Yellow Pages is my choice but people on the small side will just need a couple of paperbacks), with your knees bent at slightly more than a right angle and your hands resting gently on your torso just below your ribs. Let your elbows rest on the floor

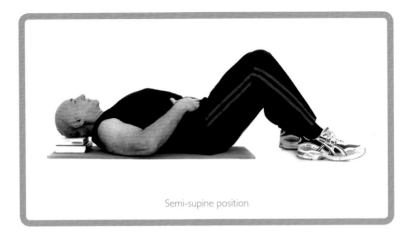
Semi-supine position

and ensure your neck is not in contact with the headrest, only the very back of your head. Preferably remove footwear and ensure your feet are flat against the floor. Try to develop a deep breathing pattern, with your jaw relaxed, to prevent tension.

Lying down in this fashion for 10-20 minutes a day will gradually help remove tension from your body, especially the neck muscles, where so many of us, as we age, start to feel tight, myself included.

There is no mystery about the Alexander Technique, it is simply a way of improving your posture and helping you to relax yet stay focused. A six-lesson course at my local Adult Learning Institute costs £21, or if you are 60 plus, £11, which I consider to be good value for money.

RPE Scale

This was originally referred to as The Borg Rating of Perceived Exertion (devised originally by Gunnar Borg) and is often seen numerated from 6-20. The scale I have adopted is deliberately simplified for ease of use (i.e. 1 – 10).

Level	Description of exertion
1	At rest, no exertion at all
2	Extremely light exertion, seated at desk/driving
3	Very moderate exertion e.g. strolling
4.	Walking purposefully, normal conversation possible
5	Walking briskly, conversation slightly harder
6	Walking at a fast pace, conversation hard to maintain (Heart rate 60%)
7	Very hard effort, breathing laboured, conversation strained (Heart rate 65-70%)
8	Effort so great that conversation is barely possible (Heart rate 80%)
9	Perspiring heavily, very difficult to converse (Heart rate 85%)
10	Maximum effort, only possible of maintaining for a very short spell, conversation impossible.

It is quite commonly used for monitoring anybody who is not yet ready, or averse to using a heart rate monitor (see 'Heart Rate Monitors' page 42).

How to Use the RPE Scale

It should not take too long to ascertain at which level you are working out. At least you do not need any equipment and are spared making calculations; you just need to be totally honest with yourself about how much effort you are expending. By recording your findings in a log you should be able to monitor your progress. If you keep a cardio training log you should after a time notice a reduction in perceived effort. At times like this you can step up the level of exertion in order to avoid reaching a plateau; working in the comfort zone for an extended period may achieve maintenance but is unlikely to bring about improvement.

The heart rate levels are approximated, but may prove a useful check if you decide to experiment with a heart rate monitor as stated in the heart rate monitor section (page 42). Be guided primarily by how you feel in yourself rather than by any training tools.

Apply the RPE scale to all the training you undertake from this book. Listen to your body and train safely. Get to know when to slow down or switch off.

11. Heart Rate Monitors and Heart Rate Training Zones

Why Use a Heart Rate Monitor?

Your heart rate is the most reliable indicator of how hard you are working out, and a heart rate monitor is the best tool to employ for the job. There are more complicated formulae than the one I have chosen (age deducted from 220 for men and 230 for women) but if you are a newcomer to heart monitoring I feel it is the simplest to understand and use.

How Does It Work?

An elastic belt secures in place a sealed transmitter that picks up impulses from your heart and relays that information to your wrist monitor or a compatible receiver on the training equipment you are working out on.

Getting to Grips with It

This health aid was developed by a Finnish professor of electronics, and if you get one, and start getting in too deep, you may wish you had a similar background in order to set it up. My advice is to work on a "need to know" basis; keep it basic for your specific needs and you will find it can be a terrific help for both fitness and weight management.

The inventor, Seppo Saynajakangas, marketed his early models in 1982 as Polar, his company's brand name. To this day Polar are still regarded as the number one manufacturer and it is perhaps unfortunate that most literature, written to explain and instruct the use of monitors, reads like an advertisement for Polar products. Polar models range from roughly £40 to £400 according to features, not accuracy; even modestly priced models by Polar or other makes have a high degree of accuracy.

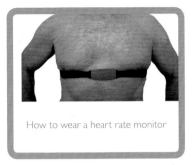
How to wear a heart rate monitor

I splashed out £39.99 on an Oregon Scientific 'Smart Trainer' and somehow managed to resist the temptation to hunt down and kill the fiend who designed the unhelpful User Manual. It does, however, do the job I bought it for – it tells me what my heart rate is while I am training.

Before you can get started you will need to enter your personal data into the monitor, including your maximum heart rate, training zone, and upper and lower heart limits. I hope the following will explain why you need them and how to determine them.

Working it out (calculator may be required)

To determine your maximum heart rate (MHR) I have used the 'Age Predicted Formula' – a rough approximation, but cost-free and accurate enough for our purpose. You simply need to deduct your age from 220 (men) or 230 (women).

Example:

If you are a man of 50 then 220 - 50 = 170 (MHR)
If you are a woman of 65, then 230 - 65 = 165 (MHR)

> To calculate your workrate zone, just work out your upper and lower limits. For example:
> A 60 year old woman on a weight management programme will need to work in the 60%-70% range.
>
> 230 - 60 = 170 (MHR)
> 170 x 60% = 102 (lower heart rate)
> 170 x 70% = 119 (upper heart rate)

So, in order to burn 85% of calories from fat while training, the lady is going to have to stay in the 102 to 119 range.

Most models will bleep if you stray from the zone (even my cheapish model does.)

How to put the monitor on

1. Hook up the transmitter to the elasticised belt. Make sure the interior is flat and the plastic connectors lie flat (rather than have them digging into your chest).

2. You know roughly where your heart lies (physically speaking), so set the transmitter across the 'nipple line' for men and just below the bra-line for women.. You can actually buy Polar bras that encompass the transmitter for £25 (ProActive Health).

3. Moisten the interior of the transmitter with water or saliva to make a better connection; to put it inelegantly – spit on it and smear it.

4. If for some reason you elect to wear the belt over the top of your clothing, then the fabric below it needs to be dampened.

5. Note the basic heart rate showing on your wrist monitor or the equipment you are about to use. Many treadmills, cycles and rowers have compatible receivers to pick up signals from your transmitter and thereby save you from repeatedly glancing at your wrist.

Levels 1 & 2

If you are unfit your resting heart rate will be high and you should not have to work excessively hard to reveal your proper training rate. Stay in this training zone until your resting heart rate is decidedly lower before moving up into the next zone.

Levels 3 & 4

If you are already fit your resting heart rate is probably low, and your training programme should be of higher intensity.

Levels 1, 2, 3 & 4

Heart rates can drop significantly from the onset of your training as you progressively become fitter, so reassess regularly (monthly would probably be a good period of time) and keep a log of your heart rate to keep tabs on your progression.

Tip

Even if you wear a heart rate monitor, continue to be governed by your own instincts regarding your well-being. Never ignore feelings of distress or breathing difficulties – ignore what the monitor tells you and STOP TRAINING! The monitor may be smart and sophisticated but it is only a machine and cannot tell you if you feel unwell – don't let it become the be-all and end-all of your training.

Heart Rate Monitor Training Zones

Heart rate intensity level	Training level
50% Moderate The "healthy heart" range	Level 1
60% Weight loss management Burns up to 85% of calories as fat	Levels 2-3
70% - Aerobic Zone Increases endurance, improves cardiovascular and respiratory systems. Burns calories as 50% fat, 50% carbohydrates	Levels 3-4
80% - Anaerobic Zone Makes substantial improvements in fitness condition. Burns calories as 85% carbohydrates, 15% fat.	Level 4
90% - Danger Zone! Elite athletes only - short bursts only, maintains superb condition.	n/a

Workout Location - Gym vs. Home

Gym	Home
Superior equipment	Train when you like
Instruction available	Hygiene to your standards
No need to set aside home space	No travel hassle or costs
No need to buy, repair or update equipment	No gym fees and no membership price rises
Social amenities	Privacy, no embarassment or comparison
No ringing doorbells or telephones, TV or music of your choice	Not subjected to off-putting or loud music to other people's tastes

12. Flexibility and Stretching

Maintaining flexibility as we get older is important. It can improve your performance with regard to physical activity as well as your day to day tasks. It should also reduce the risk of injury. Post-exercise stretches will speed your recovery from training, in addition to maintaining, or even further developing your level of flexibility.

Thus, your training should usually encompass the following phases: the warm-up, the workout, the warm-down and the warm-down stretch.

The Warm-Up

Cold muscles do not enjoy being stretched. Think of putty or plasticine before you have warmed it in your hands prior to use; if you tried to stretch it in its cold state it would simply tear. Warming-up is essential for two main reasons:

> 1. The body functions better when warm, enabling the muscles to become more pliable
>
> 2. The warm-up helps you focus and prepare mentally for your workout. It, hopefully, puts you in the mood.

Muscles at rest need only 15% of total blood flow, whereas high activity requires 80% of total blood flow as the muscles demand more fuel. The transfer of the supply cannot happen quickly, and so warm-up should be anything from 5-15 minutes, according to the individual and the intended level of exertion.

The activity should be continuous, rhythmic and (ideally) specific or relative to the workout ahead. Always ensure you wear adequate clothing to stay warm; you can always shed your outer layers as you get warmer.

To stretch or not to stretch before exercise? The debate rages; the argument revolves around the fact that stretching can leave the muscles in a state that makes exercise more difficult, in complete contradiction to the assumed logic that it makes exercise easier.

For years we were told the importance of a short pre-exercise stretch after warm-up and joint mobilisation, taking 6-10 seconds per body part. The stretch was always performed standing as it was considered that lying down or sitting would allow the body to cool, to the obvious detriment of the warm-up. Suddenly – all change! Fitness gurus seem unable to arrive at a unified agreement on this thorny subject.

So – what course to take? If you, like myself, have been doing a short stretch (total time about one minute) for years and have had no ill-effects or loss of performance (not that I'd notice much these days) my advice is to carry on regardless.

Why not experiment? Try skipping the short stretch and see if it makes any discernible difference. The sports physiology community changes opinions at such a dazzling pace; I confidently expect it to change in a short time with regard to this subject.

Short Stretch

(All stretches are performed while standing in the 'short stretch')

Shoulders, back, chest,

Hamstrings, quads, calves, Achilles/ soleus.

This stretch should be followed by mobility exercises for shoulders, knees, ankles and neck.

Warm-down stretch

One point all fitness professionals will agree upon is that the optimal time for stretching is after your workout, when the muscles are blood-enriched, warm and therefore pliable. It will help to speed your recovery, reduce muscular soreness and begin the process of waste clearance.

During exercise, lactic acid and other by-products build-up to a greater or lesser extent – depending on the individual and how much you have exerted yourself. So, after your workout it is essential to warm down as this (amongst other benefits) also helps to clear lactic acid and reduce muscle soreness. Anyone who has ever suffered from the dreaded D.O.M.S. (delayed onset muscle soreness) will appreciate the wisdom of avoiding this particular form of agony by a warm-down and a good stretch. This is when you can lay down on your mat and hold those stretches, now that your warm muscles and ligaments are in a receptive state.

The Stretches

You can avail yourself of any number of books on flexibility, which vary in how much technical information and detailed instruction they provide. I have worked on the basis that for now what you need to know is:

1. Which muscles to stretch

2. How to stretch them

I prefer a system whereby I start at the shoulders and work down, making a return trip to finish off with the neck stretch, which I consider the most important as so many people retain stress and tightness here. For this reason I have added extra neck stretches.

If you feel inflexible, try not to settle for it by consoling yourself with such excuses as: "it's my age" – you can improve your flexibility, or at least protect what you have if you stretch regularly; "I've never been flexible" – then there's no time like the present to improve.

Get into a habit of stretching on a daily basis. Have an abbreviated stretch as soon as you get out of bed, it may spare you from hobbling or limping on the journey to the bathroom. But be careful as this is the time when your muscles are likely to be at their least pliable as they've been out of action all night!

Just have a stretch session

The warm-down stretch can be used as a stand-alone session, just so long as your muscles are warm before you start. Consider taking up Yoga, Tai Chi, Pilates or The Alexander technique if you want to improve your posture as well as your flexibility.

It must be considered that weight training will improve your strength, but not your flexibility, which is an equally important aspect of your well-being; so many people have a good weights workout but neglect to stretch properly afterwards.

Flexibility is the best example of the maxim: *Use it – or lose it!*

Ballistic stretching

Ballistic stretching involves bouncing, jerky movements making it highly inadvisable, as the movement lacks the required control and does not allow the muscles to stretch adequately. Taken to the extreme it can cause soreness and even injury. Best left as the premise of finely tuned athletes, supervised by experienced coaches.

Stretch slowly! No bouncing please!

Emphasising the point made above – make your stretching slow and leisurely. Never force it or hurry it.

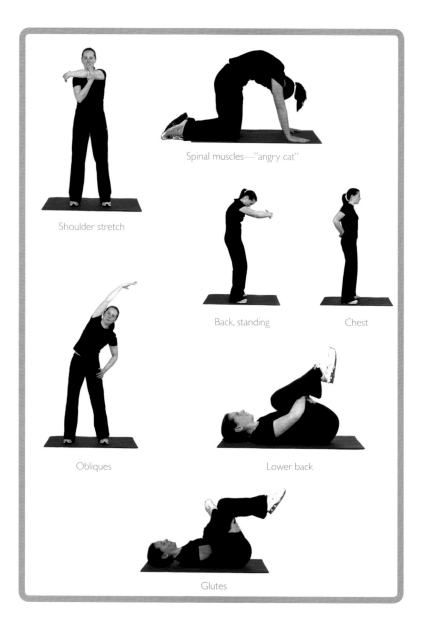

Shoulder stretch

Spinal muscles—"angry cat"

Back, standing

Chest

Obliques

Lower back

Glutes

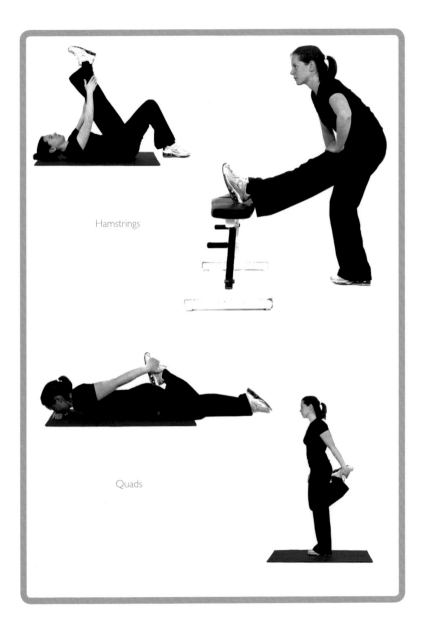

Hamstrings

Quads

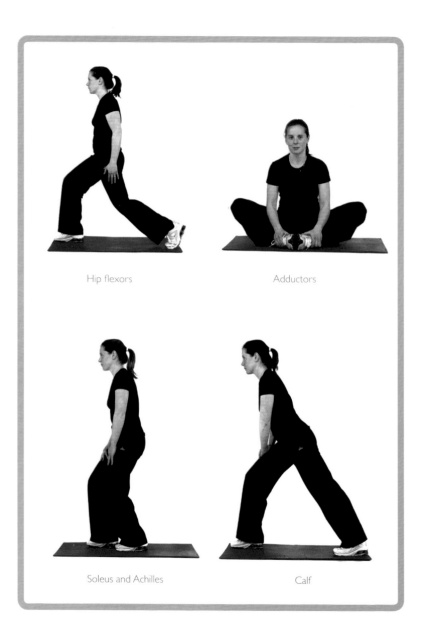

Hip flexors

Adductors

Soleus and Achilles

Calf

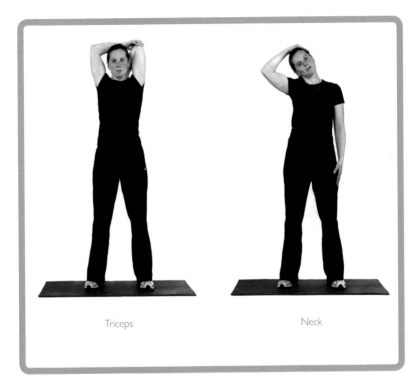

Triceps   Neck

13. Abdominal and Core Training

If you are looking to protect and strengthen your back the best place to start is not at the back, but at the front. Your abdominal muscles, especially the deep-lying ones, help form a solid corset for your back. People with an inordinately protruding stomach do not usually have stomach pain, but back pain, as their spine battles to pull up something the size and weight of a holiday-makers suitcase. Working your abs is the key to giving your back a sporting chance, as well as improving your posture (bad posture is a common cause of back pain).

As we age it takes us longer to recover from falls but a strong mid-section provides a powerful base to give stability when balance is threatened by demanding movements, both those you may make involuntarily and those imposed upon you by external factors. Nevertheless, statistics show that falls and older people are a worrying combination.

> "A significant problem in elderly people that can lead to morbidity, mortality and loss of independence is falls.
>
> (Morris and Shoo, "Exercise and Physical Activity in Older People".)

Don't bother to look up 'morbidity' – it so depressed the hell out of me, I went off to do some more crunches.

Apart from the health-threatening factors is the matter of how we look. It is not just younger people who want to look good in a swimming costume; people of all ages usually have some image consciousness and pride in their appearance. A mid-section that overflows the waistband or has the consistency of watery jelly needs to be dealt with by a two-pronged attack. The first prong is a close examination of dietary intake; all the exercise in the world will count for little if there is an excessive amount of calories being consumed. It is depressing to learn that a 20-minute run uses 200-240 calories, but a Sainsbury's individual apple pie contains 220 calories. Your second prong is exercise which, of course, has the benefit of improving your fitness and health.

The question of image cannot be understated. I have not met anybody yet who has informed me they are highly satisfied with the way their spare tyre overflows their skirt or trousers. Pride in appearance and the matter of image is not exclusive to the younger generation. That being said, the superficial appearance of the abdomen remains secondary to what lies beneath. Gaining a strong, solid core supercedes the washboard look. A flat stomach does not always mean the abdominal muscles are strong – genetics play a strong hand in how your mid-section looks.

Sadly it is not possible to 'spot reduce'; working like a Trojan on one particular area of the body will not strip away fat from that area. The aim has to be for all-over reduction.

Try to concentrate on building a stabilising belt to support your back, improve your balance and posture. If you finish up with a set of abs that resemble an ice-cube tray – well, that's a bonus.

The abdominal muscles are categorised into four major divisions. We are going to look at exercises to work all of them.

Names and Functions of Main Abdominal Muscles

1. Tranversus Abdominus (transverse): constricts abdominal contents, compresses abdomen.

2. Abdominus rectus: gives support at front of the body to the lumbar spine, holds rib cage and pubis together.

3. & 4. External and Internal obliques: allows the trunk to bend forward, twist around and bend sideways.

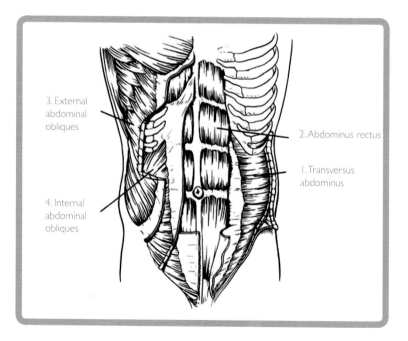

The Exercises

Remember sit-ups? You do? Well, forget them – the following will be less demanding (generally) and more beneficial.

Use a comfortable mat for all exercises that stipulate lying down. It is futile to 'tough it out' on a hard surface.

In exercises involving a Fit-Ball, ensure the ball is of the "burst-proof" variety (for obvious reasons) and that it can bear your weight. The balls come in 55, 65 and 75cm sizes. Judge the size you require by your height and weight. I personally feel it pays for tall, heavy-built guys to spend a little more if buying for the home.

The following exercises work the rectus abdominus (abs).

1. Curl-ups

All levels

Straight-leg sit-ups are inadvisable these days (unless you have a strong "core") and are definitely detrimental to the older exerciser, given the potential for harm. Instead use the version called 'curl-ups'.

These are performed with legs bent at the knee and only the shoulder blades being lifted, slowly and under control, from the floor as the trunk curls forward. Do not pull on the head or neck, and try to contract the abdominal muscles as you execute the move. If you are a newcomer to this form of exercise, try this version which suits Levels 1 and 2.

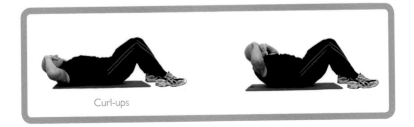

Curl-ups

Place palms of hands on thighs, slide hands up towards the knee until your shoulder blades come off the floor. Once this becomes easy, move on to placing your hands either side of your head, fingertips only making contact. Don't hold your breath!

Level 1 and 2 may prefer to start out by using an abs cradle. The advantage of the cradle is that it encourages good form and stops the user coming up too far or putting undue pressure on the neck, which is ideal for inexperienced exercisers.

2. Curls on the Fit-Ball

Levels 2 and 3

Performing your curl-ups on the Fit-Ball makes it that little more challenging. The instability of the surface increases the amount of muscle and motor skills you will recruit to execute curl-ups slowly, in a controlled movement. Keep your lower back on the ball as you rise to and fro as you would in the standard curl-up.

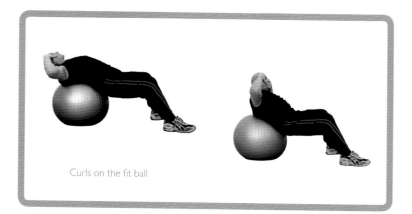

Curls on the fit ball

3. Weighted curls on the fit ball

Levels 3 and 4

As above but hold a medicine ball to your chest to give a little more resistance. If you do not have a medicine ball hold a 4-5kg dumb-bell, or a 5kg weights plate.

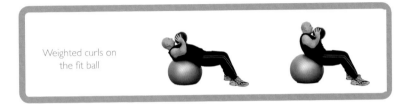

Weighted curls on the fit ball

4. Crunches

Levels 3 and 4

You can either a) place your feet up on a box, or b) bend your legs in a right angle at the knees, cross your ankles and hold them there. Then from either a) or b) curl your trunk towards your knees by only raising the shoulder blades, contracting your abs as you do so. Fingertips rest against the side of the head.

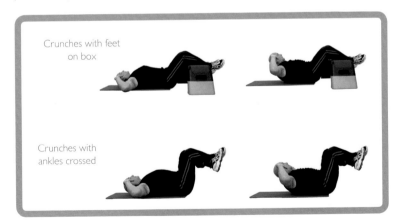

Crunches with feet on box

Crunches with ankles crossed

5. Reverse curls

All levels

Lie on your back with your hands close to your sides. Your legs should form a right angle at the knee and be crossed at the ankles, with your feet in the air. From this position slowly lift your backside off the floor by bringing your legs towards your rib cage. Once your backside has left the floor lower it back slowly to the start position. Try not to just roll backwards but contract your abs while breathing naturally. The aim is to contract your lower abdominals

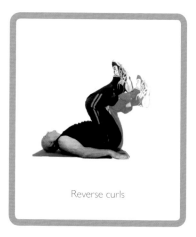

Reverse curls

rather than just move your legs in the air – they should move as a result of your abs working.

Levels 3 and 4

Lie on your back with bent legs but the soles of your feet pointing at the ceiling. Lift backside off the floor and slowly return it to the floor, contracting your abs and breathing naturally.

6. Double Crunch

Levels 3 and 4

Lie on your back with legs bent at a right angle, ankles crossed and feet in the air. Fold your arms across your chest, then bring the head and the knees toward one another.

7. Hanging leg raise

Levels 3 and 4 only

Take an overhand grip on the chin-up bar, facing outward (away from the wall). Take a deep breath and then lift your knees up to form a right angle (level 3) or to the chest (level 4). Exhale as you return to the straight leg position. Perform slowly and try to control movement in order to prevent swinging to and fro.

8. Abs Crunch Machine

Level 2, 3 and 4

Versions of these are usually found in gyms and are solidly built with pads or a bar which is pushed forward and down to allow the user to 'crunch/curl' from a seated position. Most versions allow for varying weight resistance to be applied; the Keiser version, which applies added resistance by virtue of its pneumatic technology, is about the best model I have used, as the resistance remains consistent throughout the exercise.

The following work the transversus abdominus (central muscles)

1. The kneeling plank

Level 1 and 2

Kneel on the floor, resting on your elbows. Now, while breathing easily concentrate on pulling your navel area in, and holding it for 10 seconds (count one thousand, two thousand and so on). Continue until you can achieve 30 seconds and then attempt the full exercise, detailed below.

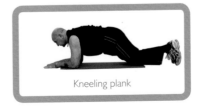

Kneeling plank

2. The Plank (also known as "The Bridge" and "Hovers")

Levels 3 and 4

Rest on your elbows and the balls of your feet. Keep your body perfectly straight with the head in line with the spine, horizontal to the floor. Hold this position rock steady as you concentrate on the navel area, pulling it in, and keeping it held in. Start with a 10 second period and gradually build up to 30 seconds and more. Try to check your form in a mirror or ask somebody to check if you are in a straight line. Be careful not to let your bottom dip as this can put extra strain on the lower back – instead, try to tilt your pelvis down towards the floor a little, which will help the correct posture.

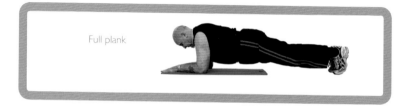

Full plank

2. Plank on the Fit-Ball

Level 4

As above but now with your feet resting on the Fit-Ball and arms extended, fingers splayed for a steady base. Contract the abdominal zone but breathe normally. Start out with 10-15 seconds then build up to 30 seconds and beyond.

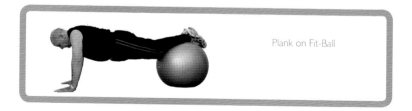

Plank on Fit-Ball

To stretch the transverse post-exercise, relax backward over the Fit-Ball

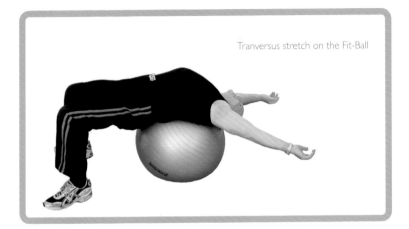

Tranversus stretch on the Fit-Ball

Obliques

1. Standing Twists

All levels

Hold a 3-5kg medicine ball (a 3-5kg dumb bell will suffice if you do not have a medicine ball) out in front of your chest with arms extended, but relaxed. Place your feet shoulder-width apart and have a slight bend in the knees to keep the legs relaxed. Aim for a complete absence of tension in this exercise. While facing to the front, keeping your hips square, turn your trunk (not your shoulders), with arms extended in a half-circle. Return to the start position before turning in the opposite direction. Do not make continuous rotations through 180 degrees – it is not healthy for your back. Always return to the start before making another turn.

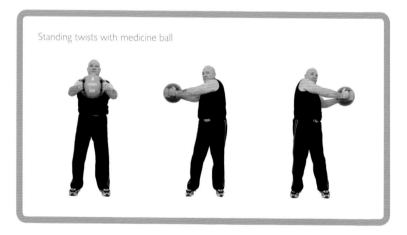

Standing twists with medicine ball

2. Russian Twists

Level 4 only

This calls for a similar rotation technique to the standing version, but with the added difficulty of stabilisation. Place your shoulders on the Fit-Ball and spread your feet apart for a solid base. As before, semi-rotate in both directions, returning to the start position before the next rotation.

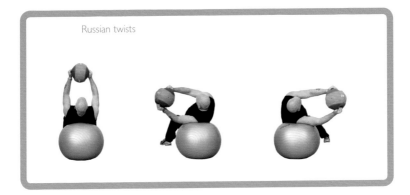

Russian twists

3. Lateral curls

Level 3 and 4

Lay sideways on or against the Fit-ball, your lower arm in contact with the ball and your legs split a bit to assist balance.

Slowly and under control lift your trunk away from the ball, pause and repeat for 10 repetitions, repeat on the other side.

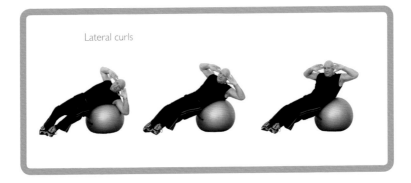

Lateral curls

4. Throwback twist.

Levels 3 and 4

This exercise needs a bouncy medicine ball and a strong flat surface (e.g. the wall of the gym or a garage). A 2-3kg ball is adequate for this manoeuvre. Stand with your back to the wall, feet shoulder-width apart. Turn and toss the ball against the wall and catch the rebound, then turn to repeat the move on the other side. Start out slowly; performing the exercise with a football is a good introduction to the exercise, progressing to a medicine ball. As you become more competent, get into a rhythm as you turn from side to side and pick up speed.

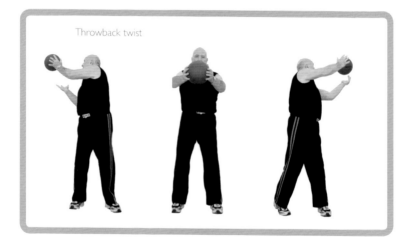

Throwback twist

5. Oblique crunch

Levels 2, 3 and 4

Lie on your back with legs bent at the knees, your feet 12"-15" in front of your backside. Raise one shoulder up and around towards the opposite knee, keeping the lower back on the floor (if you find this tricky try tilting your pelvis upwards and pushing your lower back into the mat). Return to your start position and then repeat on other side. Perform moves in a slow, controlled manner.

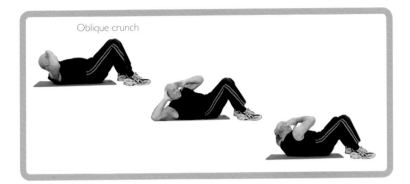
Oblique crunch

6. Dumbbell side bends

All levels

Stand with feet roughly less than shoulder-width apart, holding a 3-5kg dumbbell in your hand, arms by your side. Place the empty hand by your side, and bend your trunk to that side, keeping the hips square. Return to the start position and then repeat the move. After ten repetitions change the dumbbell over to the other hand and repeat the exercises on that side.

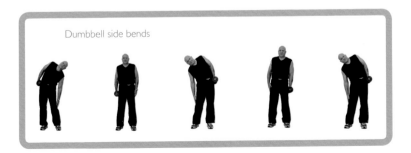
Dumbbell side bends

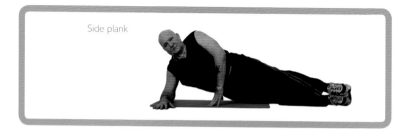

Side plank

7. The Side Plank

Level 3 (modified) and Level 4

The only contact with the ground will be the side of your feet and your bent elbow. This lateral flexion exercise is a little demanding and short spells are preferable when you first attempt it. The body should remain perfectly in line from top to toe. Breathe naturally, do not hold your breath.

Level 3:

Rest your other hand in front of you for balance and some light support before graduating to

Level 4:

Rest other hand on your hip, or by your side.

Try to build up to 30 seconds or more, then switch sides.

8. "Broomstick" twists

You may have seen people at the gym doing these, or even been advised to yourself. Hold a wooden pole, similar to a broomstick, across your shoulders and twist from side to side. This exercise was judged to be somewhere between 'dodgy' and 'downright dangerous' for quite some time by health and fitness professionals, as full rotation can prove injurious to the spine. A modified version, where the user halts at the centre, performing 'half-rotations', would be acceptable, but I feel the oblique exercises mentioned above are less restricting and altogether safer.

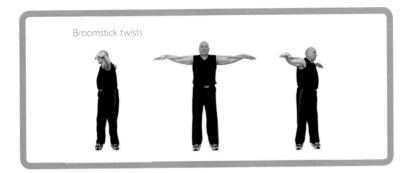

Broomstick twists

Level 1 Only

The following exercises are an accessible way for unfit people to make a positive start to firming their abdominal muscles, prior to, hopefully, progressing to the more demanding core training exercises.

1. Back Flatteners

Lie on your back with legs bent at the knees, feet about 12"-15" in front of your backside. These can be done in bed providing you have a very firm mattress!

While lying on your back feel the natural hollow of your lower back below the upper back and your backside. Now contract your abdomen to 'close the gap' as you flatten your back against the floor. Imagine you are pulling your navel deep into your stomach area. Breathe naturally, don't hold your breath.

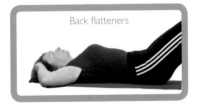

Back flatteners

Start with 10 repetitions (1 set). Progress until you can complete 3 sets of 10 repetitions without difficulty, then attempt easy version curl-ups.

2. Seated leg raise

For this exercise you need a solidly built 'carvers' chair (one with strong wooden arms). Sit in the chair in such a manner that your back is supported and your legs are bent at the knee. Grasp the arms of the chair and slowly lift your legs up towards your trunk; even a lift of a few inches will be a good start. Doing this exercise on a chair with no arms, holding the side of the chair seat is an alternative but is much more demanding. Once you become comfortable with this version, make an attempt at reverse curls.

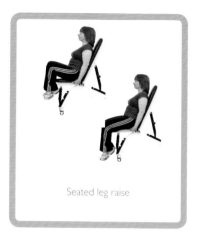

Seated leg raise

3. Easy Curls

Lay on your back with legs bent at the knee, feet about 12"-15" in front of your backside. Fold your arms across your chest, slowly raise your head far enough to see your knees, then return your head to the floor, slowly and under control – no jerkiness! Let 'slow and smooth' be your mantra.

As soon as these become tolerably easy progress to 'curl-ups' (page 59).

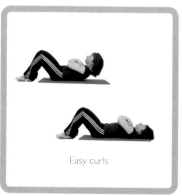

Easy curls

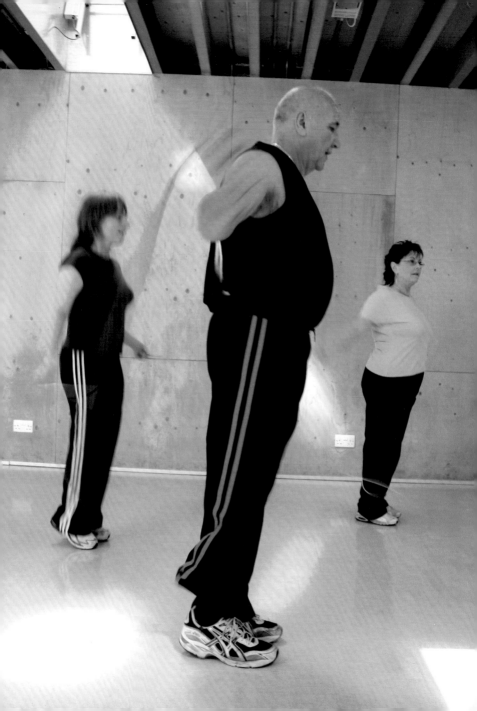

14. Press-ups and other Calisthenics

Body resistance exercises have been around as long as exercise in a structured form has been in existence. It is one of a number of such exercises which come under the heading Calisthenics, from the Greek (they liked to exercise) words 'kallos' (beauty) and 'stenos' (strength). Performed correctly, I can guarantee they will give you strength; if they make you feel, or look, beautiful, then that will be a bonus, and nothing to do with me.

If you want good conditioning then press-ups can play an integral part in your training. They work the chest, the front of the shoulders and the triceps (back of the arm) without the use of equipment, meaning (within reason) you can do them anywhere. They are invariably used in fitness tests (e.g. how many can you do in a minute) as they are a good guide to your personal strength and fitness.

When I was training a 50 year old man, I asked him how many press-ups he thought he could do. He replied, "None, I can't do them." When I asked him to try to do just one or two I discovered the reason why: his technique was dire and he was making it harder than it needed to be. With a little adjustment here and there he still only managed five repetitions but at least he now had a base to work from, which is all anybody needs. Perhaps your first shaking and trembling efforts will yield only one or two, no matter, just look to add one or two a week. I will not deny they are hard but once you get in the zone you can really surprise yourself with how many you can do.

They are best performed slowly with regular breathing, exhaling on the lifting phase – the effort.

Body weight + gravity = hard work

What should be remembered with press-ups (and most calisthenics) is that you are lifting your body weight against gravity. If I did the same action standing in front of a brick wall and pressed forward and backward I could, as could anybody, do hundreds of repetitions; when I do the same action on the floor, it becomes a very different story – I now have to work against gravity.

How many?

I feel the following will be a reasonable guideline for the over-50's. I know that many fit over-50's can match or even surpass the amount of press-ups most youngsters could manage, but I feel these scores will provide guidelines for the average Joe or Joan.

This is not how many you can do in one minute – it is how many you can actually do.

Do not hold your breath, or over-exert yourself

This is purely an exercise to establish your starting point – not to finish you off altogether!

Level 1	Males	Fewer than 5 repetitions (full press-ups)
Level 1	Females	Fewer than 8 repetitions (half press-ups)
Level 2	Males	Fewer than 10 repetitions (full press-ups)
Level 2	Females	Fewer than 12 repetitions (half press-ups)
Level 3	Males	Fewer than 20 repetitions (full press-ups)
Level 3	Females	Fewer than 15 repetitions (full press-ups)

If you can do more than the level 3 parameters then try the press-ups indicated 'level 4 only'.

Once you have found your level by the above scale, try the following;

Variations on a (press-up/ push-up) theme

Level 1 and 2

Start with 'box' press-ups or half press-ups (especially ladies, which I hope will not appear patronising but merely merciful, as I intended).

The weight rests on the knees. Always use a mat as your patella (kneecap) is not much bigger than the face of your wristwatch and must be cushioned from a hard surface to prevent soreness or injury.

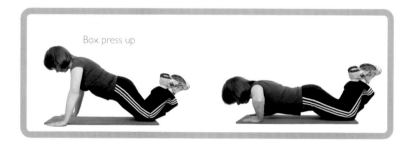
Box press up

Level 1

Build up to 3 sets of 10 repetitions with a 30 second rest between sets. Once comfortable with this, move up to level 2.

Level 2

Build up to 3 sets of 20 repetitions with a 30 second rest between sets. Once competent try full press-ups and move up to level 3.

The Full Press-up (medium width)

Level 3

Set up with body straight (dipping or bowing the body actually makes it harder), and the hands a little wider than the shoulders. Spread the fingers for a strong base. Exhale on the lifting/return phase, breathing in a controlled fashion. Do not hold your breath.

Once you can manage 20 (males) or 15 (females) without discomfort, move on to level 4.

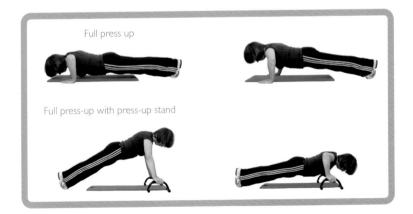

Full press up

Full press-up with press-up stand

Tip: press-up stands allow for a deeper lowering phase, but put less pressure on the wrists.

Raised feet press-up

Level 4 only

As full press-up (medium width) but with feet on raised (stable!) surface. If a bench is not handy, utilise the stairs or a strong chair. Incorporating press-up stands will increase the range of motion.

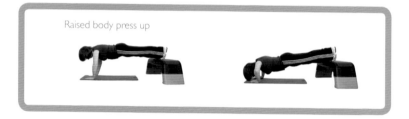

Raised body press up

The instability of the initial position makes this a harder proposition. It requires increased motor skill demands and must be performed slowly.

Fit-ball press-ups

Incline yourself towards the ball, grasping the floor with fingers spread for a solid grip, hands under shoulders. On the initial repetitions it may be wise to adopt a wide stance, which can be narrowed with confidence of execution.

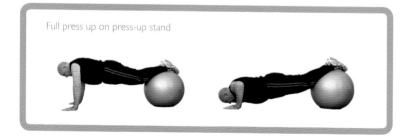

Full press up on press-up stand

Explosive press-ups

Start in the lowered press-up position, hands slightly wider than shoulders. Push up powerfully to land with your hands much wider than your shoulders. Push up again to land back in the narrower hand position; with each successive push upward, land in the former hand position.

This can be later advanced to a 'raised feet' position version.

One arm press-ups

I find this works better if you adopt a side-on wide legged stance, but there is very little that can be done to make this one easier!

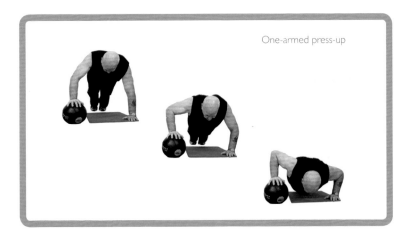

One-armed press-up

Clap hands press-ups

Most people feel like clapping once press-ups are finished, but with this variation you clap following an explosive push up before your downward descent.

Press-Ups vs. Bench Press

If press-ups are such a good workout for the same muscle group as those exercised in the bench or chest press, why do we need to do them? The difference is the press-up enables you to push up the same weight (that of your own body). Once you become competent at this and do more repetitions you are doing endurance training as opposed to strength training and only maintaining your strength. Such is the limitation of the press-up.

To get more resistance into your press-ups get a (trusted) friend to place the palm of their hand between your shoulder blades to give added weight and difficulty. Alternatively wear an evenly distributed, weighted backpack, filled with books; after twenty or more reps with this on you will begin to know what is meant by *heavy reading!*

The chest press, performed on a bench, enables you to steadily increase the amount of weight you can lift and, in doing so, increase your strength accordingly. The bench press has no upper limit; its only limit is the strength of the individual.

Muscles worked in press-ups:

Pectorals major (pecs) = chest

Triceps = back of arms

Anterior deltoids = front of shoulders

More Calisthenics

(I have omitted calisthenic exercises that work the abdominal muscles as I have listed them in the 'Abdominal Training' section).

Like press-ups the following exercises have three benefits:

- They are convenient

- They are cheap (if not free)

- They work!

The drawbacks are:

- You can only lift your own body weight, and once you can perform the exercises easily you have to devise new ways to increase resistance, such as changing the angle of the body to work harder against gravity.

Doing the Legwork

A 5 minute warm-up and short stretch, at least of the leg muscles, should precede any of the following exercises.

Step-ups

If you do not have a regular step box (e.g. Reebok Step) then improvise with a sturdy milk crate, stout wooden box or the bottom stair. Make sure the landing foot is placed fairly and squarely on the surface, be it box or floor. Either do ten steps off each foot or alternate feet for a pre-specified time.

Squats

As performed in weight training but as a weight-free exercise (also a good introduction for performing the same exercise with weights). Start with your feet shoulder-width apart and arms forward for balance when you first start.

Keep your head up and fix your eyes on a spot just above your eyeline. A

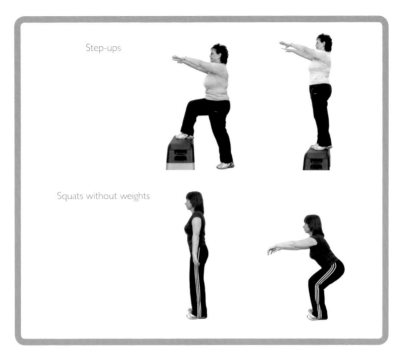

Step-ups

Squats without weights

mirror is ideal as you can check that your alignment is good. Slowly bend your knees and sink to a squatting position. Do not be dismayed if you don't sink very low; any angle you bend to will be a start in strengthening your upper leg muscles. Once you get used to the movement you may be able to increase your range.

Calf Raise

Stand on a step box, or a sturdy box, placed before a wall or window-sill. Alternatively, use your bottom stair – provided you have a handrail. This is NOT a hands-free exercise. Only once you have obtained strong hand support can you begin. Go up on your toes, pause and then lower your heels back to the box.

Level 1 and 2

This form of the exercise will be a good start for trainers at level 1 and 2 (do 10 repetitions only to begin with).

Levels 3 and 4

When you step on the box allow your heels to overhang. Drop your heels lower than the edge of the box, then go up on your toes, pause, lower heels to start position and continue.

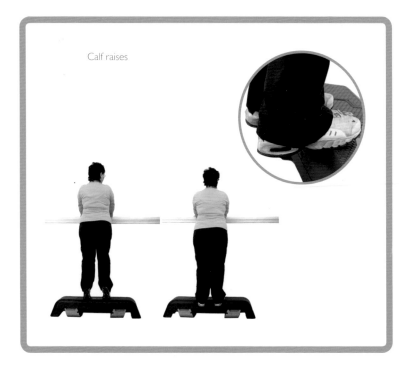

Calf raises

Lunges

Like squats, lunges are usually performed while holding weights, as a strength exercise. Without weights it is particularly beneficial for developing balance and co-ordination, combined with an endurance factor. Start with the feet shoulder-width apart. Keeping the upper body upright, step forward with one foot, bending the leg to a right angle, with the lower part of the leg vertical and the knee above the ankle (not beyond it). The rear leg should also be close to forming a right angle, with the lower leg parallel to the floor. Bring the leading leg back to the starting position and step forward with the other foot to form two right angles again. If you feel a little wobbly at first, then try spreading your arms out to the sides, like a tightrope walker, to assist your balance. Keep your head up at all times to maintain good alignment. If it is possible, check your form for good alignment in a mirror, which can be a great help.

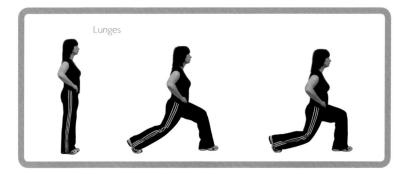

Lunges

Back Work

Back extensions

All levels

Lie face down on a comfortable surface. Remember, if it's not comfortable to start with it is hardly likely to improve after 10 repetitions. Place your hands lightly on each side of your head, fingertips only making contact and slowly lift your trunk off the floor in a slow, controlled movement. Rise up naturally; don't force the movement to gain more height.

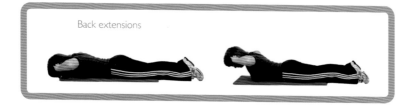

Back extensions

Chin-ups

Level 3 and 4 only

Some gyms have an assisted version of this manoeuvre, which might be a good place to start if you have not previously had the dubious pleasure of chin-ups. This is an exercise where featherweights score over heavyweights as you are lifting your own dead weight – vertically. The slim, sinewy types can usually pump out a good number of these, while the heavy built muscular types have their work cut out.

It involves gripping an overhead bar and pulling yourself high enough to look over the bar (you do not actually need to get your chin over the bar, despite the name of the exercise). It works the lats, the trapezius, teres and rhomboids, but it is in the biceps you will feel the effect, according to how much body weight you have!

There are two basic versions. Most people find version 1 slightly easier:

1. Undergrip – with hands close together

2. Overgrip – hands wide apart.

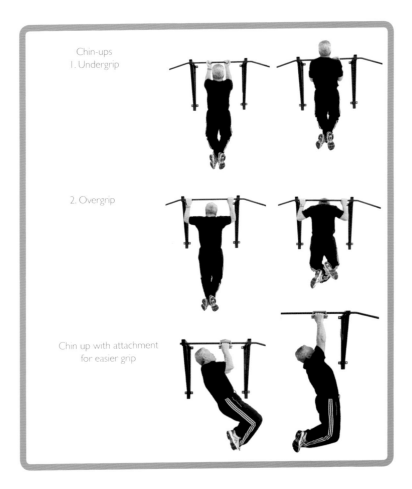

Chin-ups
1. Undergrip

2. Overgrip

Chin up with attachment
for easier grip

Tricep dips

All levels

Use a sturdy box or chair to support you. Place hands behind you with the heel of each hand firmly gripping the edge of the surface. Let your arms form a right angle, then straighten them again.

The following increase the degree of difficulty:

Level 3

Same exercise but keep legs straight

Level 4

Raise feet onto another box

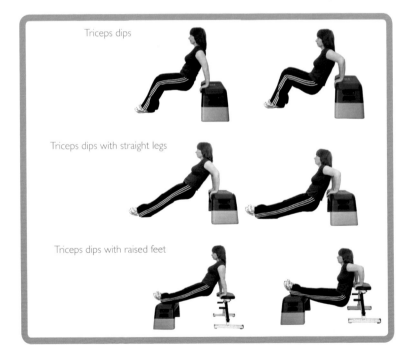

Triceps dips

Triceps dips with straight legs

Triceps dips with raised feet

15. Age and Aerobic Fitness

Rate of Aerobic Decline Per Decade

SEDENTARY	8% to 15%
ACTIVE	4% to 5%
FIT	2.5%

(Sharkey B. 2001)

The aerobic decline can be accelerated if body fat is excessive; when excess weight and body fat is controlled to acceptable levels the rate of decline can be as little as 2%.

Inactivity (a lack of aerobic exercise) will result in accelerated ageing; exercise will strengthen your heart and improve the blood supply to your muscles, reducing stiffness and putting a spring in your step.

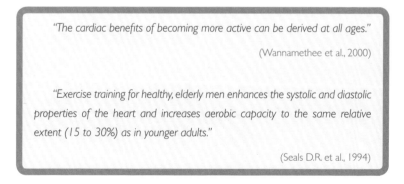

"The cardiac benefits of becoming more active can be derived at all ages."

(Wannamethee et al., 2000)

"Exercise training for healthy, elderly men enhances the systolic and diastolic properties of the heart and increases aerobic capacity to the same relative extent (15 to 30%) as in younger adults."

(Seals D.R. et al., 1994)

Anybody capable of walking is in a splendid position to enhance their fitness to a level that will keep them walking, as opposed to being wheeled around in their later years; they simply need to ensure they do as much walking as they can manage, on a daily basis (see Walking, page 90).

Report from "The New Scientist" 25th September 2004, "How to keep the spring in your heart."

Doing enough endurance exercise can keep a 70-year-old's heart as strong as one 40 years younger.

As people age, the walls of their heart stiffen, and blood enters the heart between beats. To keep pumping enough, the heart works harder, but this can result in blood backing up in the lungs, causing heart failure.

Benjamin Levine at the Presbyterian Hospital in Dallas, Texas, wanted to find out how much ageing is to blame for this kind of stiffening, compared with lack of exercise.

His team studied 24 adults approaching 70 years old. Half were past sporting champions and still averaged the equivalent of more than 50 kilometres running a week. The rest took fewer than three 30-minute sessions of exercise a week. The team compared these two groups with 14 healthy young adults around 30 years old who took as little exercise as the sedentary seniors.

As expected, the resting heart rates of the senior athletes were lower than the sedentary seniors. Surprisingly, their heart elasticity, measured as the ratio of blood pressure to the volume of blood pumped by the heart, was not only significantly higher than that of the sedentary seniors, but was almost identical to that of the sedentary juniors."

16. Walking

I find people who walk for fitness in a structured pattern tend to come from both ends of the fitness spectrum. At one extreme are those who are reasonably unfit and are starting out on a fitness plan and, at the other extreme, those who were once very fit but through various injuries can no longer run, or even jog, but can still maintain a good level of fitness through regular brisk walking.

Walking for fitness does not mean walking to the newsagents to get the Sunday morning papers instead of taking the car; it needs structure and adherence to get fit by walking. It's no good looking out the window and sighing, "Oh, it's raining, I'll leave it." Unless the weather is foul, snowy or stormy, put a waterproof on and get moving.

Footwear

Footwear is of paramount importance when you are walking any distance; that comfy pair of loafers you slip on for a stroll will not serve the purpose of the distance you are likely to cover in thirty minutes. The last thing you need as a fledgling walker are painful blisters, corns or calf pains. Not getting properly shod before you start out is a false economy. There has never been the amount of information on what is available for pain-free walking as there is at the present time. Specialist shops abound everywhere: Black's, Millet's, Field and Trek, Regatta and many more supply all leading reputable makes of footwear and apparel. You may have to consider buying a half-size bigger than you would normally wear, to allow for the fact that your feet will expand when they are hot, and if you are going to walk briskly for a good distance, they are going to get hot!

Buying shoes and socks

A few things to bear in mind when buying walking shoes and socks:

Consider what sort of terrain you will be covering, be it pavement, meadow or rocky hillsides. A specialist store will advise you accordingly.

Buy from the specialist store rather than the internet as you will need to try a few pairs on for comfort before making your final selection.

Go for shoes or boots that are lightweight and breathable.

As stated above make sure you have adequate foot room. Try to buy later in the day when, believe it or not, your feet are at their largest.

Ensure the sole is flexible. You should be able to bend it in your hand.

Wear them at home before setting off for a long hike. Good shoes do not need 'breaking in,' but it is advisable to feel comfortable in them.

Ensure the shoes don't pinch anywhere. If there is a minor irritation when you try them on in the store this will be magnified once you've gone a couple of miles in them.

Get your foot measured. Don't just say "I'm a nine."

A good assistant should be able to advise you on how to lace your shoes, according to whether you have long, narrow or broad feet.

If you have bought leather boots, treat them to a regular clean-up. Apply good quality shoe cream and allow it to soak in before buffing up. If your shoes are synthetic or a leather-synthetic combination, proof them with Nikwax or a similar product.

Buy walking socks first so you can wear them when you try your shoes on, rather than thin regular socks.

Don't throw old toothbrushes out – put them in the shoe cleaning kit box; they are great for applying cream or proofing to those 'hard to get at' sections along the welt and inside the lacing flap.

My personal favourite is to rub petroleum jelly (Vaseline) into all the stitching before stepping outdoors; in my experience the stitching usually goes first if untreated.

Socks are important. A sock that feels reasonably comfortable when you set off may harbour some nasty little seams that can chafe the tender areas of your foot and give the impression you have small stones in your shoe.

Tip – Clothing

Although it might not be the case with many new sportswear products, I would always advise against wearing a new item of clothing until it is a little "worn-in". It is usually new vests, T-shirts and, in particular, shorts that have a propensity to chafe, giving the dreaded 'runner's nipple' and the equally hideous groin or inner-leg soreness. If in doubt – smear Vaseline on the suspect areas before leaving home, or carry it with you. Be warned, I have seen these injuries serious enough to draw blood and to prove extremely distressing.

Next in order of importance is your outer coat. One that combines a waterproof outer shell and a detachable fleece is ideal, as you get two for one. Even on warm days a thin fold-up waterproof is advisable, given the vagaries of an English summer, where it is possible to combine elements of all four seasons in a single day.

Walking After Dark

Try to stay to well-lighted areas, for obvious reasons regarding the safety aspect, and invest in some reflective apparel, be it the clothing itself or strips that fasten with Velcro.

Tip - Footcare

Trim your toenails before you put your socks on, or you may find that the nail of one toe has developed an edge akin to a craft knife and has sliced into the soft skin of its neighbour. A sock soaked in blood is not an uncommon occurrence with fledgling walkers, and can leave you walking some distance in discomfort.

A blister pack is a handy item to have on board (Boots sell them, along with most 'Outdoor' shops). A small packet of plasters of various shapes and sizes is also recommended to patch up and protect painful sites en route.

Stand up when tying your laces – your foot takes up a different position in your shoe when you bend over from a seated position to lace your shoes, especially if you have raised your heel to make the job easier. So stand and place one foot on a flat surface with the foot comfortably inserted before lacing your shoes; you will be standing erect when you walk, so tie your shoes up accordingly and you shouldn't have to stop to adjust your laces.

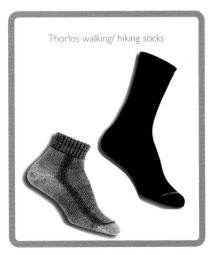

Thorlos walking/ hiking socks

Face up to it

If the forecast is for rain then you will obviously take a waterproof, but if the forecast is sunny don't forget to take sunglasses, sun cream and a lightweight hat. Sunstroke will definitely put a crimp in your outing.

Music on the Move?

If you are spending 30 minutes or more on a treadmill at the gym, facing a brick wall, a mirror or a charmless view out of the window, it's not such a bad idea to get the headphones on and listen to some music of your own, as opposed to the selection many gyms play, aimed at the average 18-25 year old taste in most cases.

If you are strolling along country footpaths well away from the traffic, you may feel the urge to listen to some suitable music to lift, or simply suit, your mood. You may want to keep up to speed with the football results, The Lions Tour or the Test Match.

Conversely, if you are walking in town or city earphones are highly inadvisable, given the risks you run of being: a) run over by not hearing an approaching vehicle while crossing the road; b) battered by one of the 'new generation' of cyclists (e.g. adults who belt along pedestrian pavements with total disregard to the safety of those on foot; c) mugged – sad to mention this but in the district of my birth and current workplace, Hackney, in East London, only a total stranger or alien would not realise they need all their senses about them. In any urban environment, forfeiting your sense of hearing is dangerous.

If you have any doubts as to wear headphones or not, always err on the side of caution.

Stretching

Many people consider that although running necessitates stretching, walking does not, as it is 'gentler' exercise. While you may not be pounding the pavement you will, nevertheless, be putting your leg muscles through a strenuous test of endurance, so look after them, especially if you want to prevent aches and pains in the days after your walk. This requires that you stretch fully, after your walk. A full set of stretches before you set off is not necessary, unless you have always done so, in which case it should do no harm as long as the muscles you stretch are warm enough – never stretch cold muscles or perform ballistic (bouncing) stretches.

Stretches and Mobilisation

Wait until your muscles are warm before you take your short stretch and mobilisation. Cold muscles lack the richly oxygenated blood of warm muscles, and must be treated cautiously. Hard stretching before starting out can be counter-productive.

> Walk for 5-10 minutes, depending on ambient temperature. A very cold day may take longer for you to feel slightly warm..
>
> Loosen up the joints, rotate ankles (just a few ankle rolls).
>
> Circle arms to loosen shoulders (slowly but powerfully).
>
> Lift your upper leg until it is parallel, or nearly parallel, with the ground to get your hips mobilised.
>
> Raise upper leg behind you to 90 degrees or more and allow to swing gently forward to mobilise knees.
>
> Stretch calf muscles by standing an arm's length from the wall and, keeping heels on the floor, take your head to the wall until you feel the gentle stretch in the back of your lower leg.

All of the above should be done within a few minutes or the body will lose its heat, and for the same reason try to keep up a good tempo to avoid cooling down too much.

The Benefits of Walking for Fitness

(based on regular 30 minute brisk walk)

1. Reduces blood pressure

2. Tones leg muscles

3. Improves cardiovascular endurance

4. Lowers cholesterol

5. Increases metabolism, thereby burning more calories

6. Removes distractions (if you turn your mobile phone off) and helps you think clearly. A recent study in The New Scientist claims that even a sedate walk for half an hour three times a week can improve your powers of concentration by up to 15%.

7. Suits older adults, especially those with arthritis, as it has a lower injury rate than sports participation.

Boost Your Walking Power

When it comes to the actual biomechanics of walking, with regard to the older person, two-thirds of their body mass (the head, arms and trunk) need good balance control to ensure good walking posture. The hip area needs strength when the hip is extended during walking and some exercise to assist this is highly beneficial.

If you don't want to take on a full strength weights or bodyweight plan from other sections of this book, it might still benefit you to do a few exercises to strengthen the hip and upper leg region (see suggested exercises on the next page).

The Programmes

I have split the schedule in two: one for those training at the gym and another for the 'outdoor' walker.

I have allotted slightly lesser times for levels 1 and 2 at the gym, as they may have to familiarise themselves with the treadmill and I do not want to put any pressure on them at this tender stage!

AT THE GYM

Level 1

Set the treadmill to a comfortable pace and aim for a target time of merely 5 minutes. This should be attainable by everybody who managed to arrive at the gym under their own steam!

Each session you undertake after this, build up in two minute increments, until you get up to 15 minutes, which should be session 6. Once you can manage 15 minutes comfortably, step it up to 5 minute increments every other session – but I must stipulate it should be performed comfortably.

Session	1	2	3	4	5	6	7	8	9	10	11	12
Minutes	5	7	9	11	13	15	20	20	25	25	30	30

Once you have reached 30 minutes try to increase the pace, minimally at first. Use the RPE scale (page 40) to see how you feel and how much effort you have applied, or check on your heart rate monitor, if you have one (see HRM page 46). On the RPE you should be at around 3 at first, rising to 5.

The advantage of using the treadmill (apart from the obvious – not getting wet, or treading in anything, and so on) is that you will be able to tell how many calories you have burned (try not to expect too much here – the machine's calculations are not likely to be up to NASA standard) and how far you have travelled. Make a note of the distance and attempt to improve on it, however minimally, with each successive session. Try not to go below 2 mph on the machine's speedometer after you pass the 5 minute mark.

Level 2

Similar to the above but start at 10 minutes and then increase your times by 5 minutes on alternate sessions, until you reach 30 minutes comfortably.

Session	1	2	3	4	5	6	7	8
Minutes	10	15	15	20	20	25	25	30

Once you have reached 30 minutes attempt to beat your previous time for this distance. Try not to go below 2.5 mph on the machine's speedometer.

Levels 3 & 4

Start at 20 minutes then increase by 5 minutes each session to 30 minutes. Use the speedometer on the treadmill to ensure you keep your speed up, try not to drop below 3 mph once you have gone past the 5 minute mark. Once a week try to complete a 45 - 60 minute walk, (so long as other gym users don't become abusive about you hogging the machine).

Level 4

Consider holding 1.5-2kg hand weights to increase resistance.

Levels 2, 3 and 4 should refer to the RPE scale and compare it to previous efforts. Many machines are compatible with Heart Rate Monitors, and if you do not have one of your own ask if you can loan one; the signal from the chest belt is picked up and displayed by the machine to save you from constant glancing at your wristwatch.

The Outdoor Walker

If the benefits of walking on a treadmill at the gym are: dry conditions, convenience, no protective clothing required and, for many, lack of embarrassment, then the benefits of walking outside far outweigh these. Consider these:

Clean fresh air (as long as you are not walking alongside a major motor road).

No television or blasting music (both of someone else's choice).

Scenery (30 minutes of looking at a brick wall or the same view out of a window can be less than inspirational).

If you want to get more out of your walk carry a backpack (handy for water and so on) as added resistance; I've yet to see anyone on the treadmill with a backpack on. I have, however, heard them bleating into their mobile phone at full volume (you should be spared from this ordeal).

The downside, of course, is the chance of getting caught in a heavy downpour, so carry waterproof clothing in the backpack if the weather looks dubious.

In The Backpack / Daypack

Water

Light snack (apple, dried fruit or nuts)

Lipsalve

Plasters or blister pack

High factor suncream

Tissues (especially in the winter) and medicated wipes

Waterproofs

Hat with a peak or brim

Clean pair of socks

Possibly a small hand towel

This kit should see you set for a long walk, with an air of confidence that you are prepared for anything. With all that stuff on your back as added resistance you'll be assured of a decent workout too!

A daypack is a little larger and roomier, and usually has a front strap to stop the pack bouncing about on your back. Day packs usually have superior padding to most backpacks and sit easier on the back.

Good quality waterproof trousers are a decent investment: lightweight, offering UV protection, yet breathable. Zip-off lower legs can suit our unpredictable climate in helping you cool off on warm days. Fabrics improve all the time and this is a highly competitive market where bargains can be found. If your favourite trousers are an essential item, but you don't want them caked in mud, consider packing up a pair of gaiters – lightweight elasticated sleeves to cover your lower legs in mud, snow or puddles.

Tip

Carry a £10 or £20 note in case you are injured and need to pay for transport to take you home. While it may be easier in the city to hail a taxi, it is still preferable in less built-up areas to wait ages for a bus than to hobble home in agony, aggravating your injury. For the same reason carry your mobile in case you need to summon help.

Suggested exercises for walking

Floor hip extensions

Bridging

Floor hip adduction

Squats

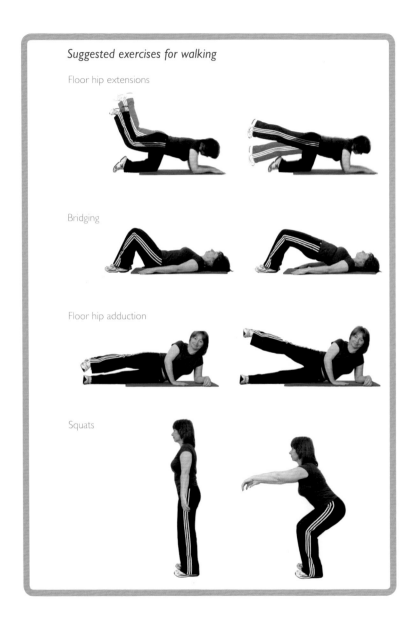

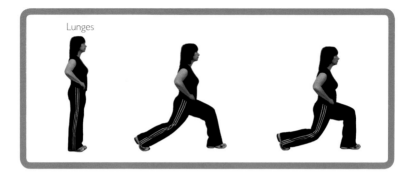
Lunges

Getting started

It will help to have some landmarks on your route, possibly a tree, a lamppost, a street or park sign. Whether you are setting off from your street door or from somewhere in parkland, a significant landmark to head for will help to chart your progress and assist you in stepping up the pace a little on each successive workout.

Tip - surface

You may have little or no choice in this matter but, if you can, seek out sandy paths, tarmac or firm grass surfaces. They will all prove kinder than stone or pavement.

Tip - pedometers

On the workout below there will come a stage when I will ask you to try to increase the distance you will walk. A pedometer is handy for this purpose.

Level 1

Week 1

Shod in comfortable shoes and socks, wearing a wristwatch, set off on your maiden walk aiming at 5 minutes out, turn around, and 5 minutes back home. Aim to do this for 5-6 days of your first week (RPE 3-4)

Week 2

Aim for a 15 minute round trip on 5-6 days this week (RPE 4-5).

Week 3

Step it up to 20 minutes on 5-6 days (RPE 4-5).

Week 4

Increase to 25 minutes on 5-6 days (RPE 4-5).

Week 5

Increase to 30 minutes on 5-6 days (RPE 4-5).

You have reached your target time. Your next progression is to see if, in covering this distance, you can walk a little faster and therefore progress further on your route in the allotted time.

Week 6

Remain on 30 minutes but for 6 days a week and rest on 7th (RPE 5-6).

After a further four weeks of this move up to Level 2.

Level 2

Week 1

Aim for a 15 minute walk for 5-6 days (RPE 4-5).

Week 2

Increase to 20 minutes for 5-6 days (RPE 4-5).

Week 3

Increase to 25 minutes for 5-6 days (RPE 4-5).

Week 4

Increase to 30 minutes for 5-6 days (RPE 4-5).

Week 5

Increase to 30 minutes for 6 days and rest on the 7th day (RPE 4-5).

Week 6

As above but now try to increase the distance you can cover in 30 minutes and aim to complete a 45 minute walk once a week (RPE now 5-6).

After this progress to level 3 and 4 workout, coming in at week 2.

Levels 3 and 4

Week 1

Start at a moderate pace for 30 minutes on 5-6 days of your first week (RPE 4-5).

Week 2

Increase the distance you covered in the first week by walking more briskly for 30 minutes, with one walk of 45 minutes (RPE 4-5).

Week 3

Increase to 45 minutes, of varied pace, for 5-6 days (RPE 4-6).

Week 4

Increase to 60 minutes, of varied pace, for 5-6 days.

Week 5

Walk for 60 minutes 5-6 days a week. Try to increase the distance you cover by stepping up your pace.

Week 6

Walk for 60 minutes for 3 days and for 120 minutes once a week. Try to include uphill gradients, which will help to improve your strength and stamina.

After week 6, levels 3 and 4 should set out their own structure for training, perhaps investigating "power walking" or interspersing their walks with days designated to a jogging workout. Changing your routine will prevent boredom setting in; keep looking for new routes and schedules to keep your training fresh.

The Indoor Walker

If you are using a treadmill at home then use the gym workout as listed above (page 97). If you are considering buying a treadmill in order to train at home make a reasoned judgement on which machine will best suit your needs. Space and weight are considerations – you don't want to plunge through the ceiling or get it home only to discover you can't get it up the stairs, or through the front door. Cost is another story altogether, although you can find second-hand treadmills. The photo here shows a top-of-the-range Life Fitness treadmill. I think it is generally recognised that quality machinery in this respect does not come cheaply and you usually get what you pay for.

17. Running and Jogging

What's the difference? As I see it jogging is slow running, or running in a relaxed easy style, or merely one form of running, as is 'sprinting'. For the purposes of this chapter I have referred to it as 'running', but substitute 'jogging' if that's the way you see it. I used to tell people "I run", but catching my reflection in a large plate glass window as I loped listlessly through an industrial estate, I would have to now admit, "I jog".

Running can benefit both aerobic and anaerobic systems, but for Levels 1 and 2 we will be staying purely in the aerobic region, especially if you are a newcomer to running. At this stage it is only fair to warn you – it can become addictive.

The Benefits

Improves heart, lungs and muscle strength and tone.

Burns fat.

Reduces stress.

Protects against osteoporosis.

Suits people of all ages.

Before you start

There are some important considerations before you go bounding down the street or around the park that you should be aware of:

Shoes

Runners need running shoes; those comfortable old Green Flash tennis shoes just won't do. We need to get specific here in order to avoid the agonies that lie in wait for the ill-shod runner.

Purchase your shoes from a recommended, good quality running shop, such as Runners Needs, Run and Become or other specialist outlets. Try not to scrimp on your shoes; you will be glad you didn't. You may have to travel a few miles to find a specialist running shop but it will be well worth the trip. I would always advise going to a shop as opposed to buying by mail order or online, as fitting is an essential part of the purchase. Most of the reputable shops can be located via their advertisements in magazines such as *Runner*, *Runner's World* and *Masters Athletics*; these magazines also regularly test and make recommendations on shoes and give great tips on all aspects of running.

When fitting your shoes, the retailers will usually get you to run on a treadmill and video your gait to see what kind of style you have, this is standard practice at Runners Needs. He or she will probably tell you that you *pronate*, *supinate* or are *normal*. Whichever they detect will govern their choice of shoe to suit your individual needs. The retailers are runners themselves and fully understand the importance of getting you off on the right track. They hope to see you return time and time again for a new pair as you wear your shoes out in your new-found enthusiasm!

Some shoes use gel capsules in the heel, the forefoot, or both; others have air capsules, kinetic wedges and all manner of rocket science-sounding materials, which is why professional advice becomes important when faced with the dazzling array of features.

Most people, once they get their new running shoes on, suddenly feel the urge to get going in them, known as *"new shoe syndrome"*. They need no wearing in, they should feel great the first time you set off in them – or, if not, take them back to the shop, they will understand if there is something awry and should, if they worry about their reputation, happily change them.

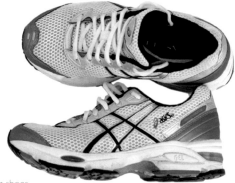

Asics running shoes

It should not be assumed, unfortunately, that even the finest footwear in the universe will save you from injuries if there is an underlying problem. As we age our feet tend to get flatter and orthotic innersoles may be required. I got a ready-to-wear version issued by the National Health Service, as individual made-to-measure pair can work out expensive. If you find you are suffering from strains and pulls, even in your comfy shoes, it might be worth contacting a specialist in sports injuries before you are laid off with an injury.

Clothing

If you are unsure of the weather (like so many of the weather forecasters appear to be in Britain) dress up rather than down. A hat can always be carried or stuffed into a pocket if you get too hot and a long-sleeved top can be tied around the waist. In winter a hat is needed to prevent heat escaping from the top of the head, where a large proportion of body heat is given off.

Thin waterproofs are a worthwhile investment. They will not only protect you from the wet, but from the wind as well. There are some great running garments available that will keep you warm, cool or wick away sweat as desired. They are usually well made and seem to last forever, as wear on them is minimal. The running magazines carry adverts for them; the web has an enormous choice and the specialist shops always have a good stock.

Your most important item of clothing, after your shoes, is your socks. Invest in running socks. They are a little more expensive than ordinary sports socks, but last a long time. Never wear nylon socks or a pair that have raised or ridged seams. They will wait until you are half way through your run and then apply their nasty little edges, ruining your run. Never wear new items (except running socks) against your skin – beware the dreaded blood-drawing runner's nipple. If in doubt, smear all potentially vulnerable areas with Vaseline. Shiny new shorts or tight nylon vests are to be steered well clear of.

That nylon replica football shirt may declare your undying devotion to Leyton Orient or Tranmere Rovers, but you would be much better off in a soft cotton t-shirt instead.

Cotton and polyester, in my opinion, are good materials when it comes to running kit. Dri-fit, Coolmax and Clima-proof are branded names for materials designed purely for training; you generally pay more but I have found they usually deliver good quality.

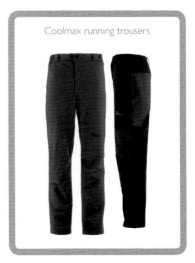

Coolmax running trousers

In summer, get running shorts made of cotton or polyester, and get track trousers for running or jogging when the weather becomes too cool for shorts. Serious participants go for Ron Hill Tracksters, which are close-fitting and purpose-made, which is why many athletes train in them. You can also get tight-fitting leggings, many in lurid designs to herald your approach; just on a personal note I prefer something a little roomy with a zip pocket for my door key.

Also to be avoided at all costs are aids such as bin-liners, intended to help you lose weight, but which will dehydrate you; fine for the first half mile of the marathon until the experienced runners get their core heat working, but dangerous for the novice runner. Leg weights, 'to strengthen the legs' are another spurious device – they ruin your running rhythm and can cause injury.

Ladies Only

Lady runners will almost certainly need a sports bra, which will also give decent support in other vigorous activities. The best-selling Dans-Ez Minimal Dance Bra provides strong straps and a 'cupless' design. It was chosen by the British armed forces as the best choice for their female troops. This is a very competitive market with new innovations being introduced all the time, so professional advice is a wise option. Ladies should remember, especially if they are newcomers to running, that their regular day-to-day bra is unlikely to support them when running and could prove painful and possibly restrict their freedom of movement.

Surfaces

If you are just starting out, look for parkland with firm grass or sandy paths as they are ideal, user-friendly surfaces. If you have, or have had, knee problems, these are definitely the surfaces for you, at least initially. Sandy beaches look inviting but are only of value if they have hard-packed sand – soft sand pulls hard on the Achilles tendon. The worst surface, sadly, is the most common and widely available: pavement, with its jarringly unforgiving concrete.

Seasoned runners simply get used to running on pavement, and learn to adapt, usually from necessity. Novices would well be advised to seek an alternative surface unless it is unavoidable.

If you live in an area of tarmaced pavements, or the communications cable-layers have recently left a soft tarmac path, count yourself fortunate; tarmac is a great surface to run on. A hypermarket car park on a summer evening (or if it's well lit) makes a reasonable jogging track. Even if the surroundings are uninspiring the surface should be favourable.

I would advise against running distances on Astroturf – it can play havoc with hamstrings in particular.

Safe and Sensible Running

It is an extremely sad indictment of our society that women runners – and in some urban areas after dark, male runners too – need extra vigilance. It is always better to err on the side of caution, and I advise the following steps for improving your safety:

> Women who run in any area in which they do not feel totally safe, should ideally find a running partner or partners.

> Leave the iPod or walkman at home if there is traffic or you know the area has a dubious reputation. I have spoken to more than one person who has suffered being mugged through inattention caused by wearing earphones. They did not hear the approach of their assailant, who was obviously aware of this fact. A high-end iPod is a tempting item to the pondlife that prey on the unsuspecting – leave it indoors and have your wits about you.

> Wear reflective materials at night; a reflective vest is advisable. A soft lightweight mesh vest, the Nathan Tri Colour vest comes with zipped

pockets and night visibility up to 1,200 feet, and costs about £20; running stores provide a wide choice of vests, ankle bands and clip-on flashing mini-lights. Run towards the traffic if you have to run in the roadside, and keep in single file, never side by side or bunched.

Beware of the dog! Keep away from dogs whose owners have let them off the leash. I speak as a former dog-owner and still a dog-lover but I've been a victim of dog assaults twice; a Dachshund nipped my ankle and a huge, friendly-looking Airedale bowled me over. Both owners, curiously, made the same remark, "Well, he's never done that before!" as if somehow I had contributed to the attack, and should be apportioned some of the blame. I also, curiously, made the same remark on both occasions, but I won't repeat it here. Give the loose hound a very wide berth.

Run in well-lit areas at night and never run through areas of darkness. I once missed the edge of the kerb in a gloomy country lane (although an area I was familiar with) and sprained my ankle. I have never run in bad light since and strongly advise you not to.

Carry a coin in case you need to phone home, or your mobile phone if it is small and light enough, in case of emergency. I got a useful tip from a fellow runner who had recently come back from injury and was concerned about a possible relapse – to carry a bank-note under the innersole of your running shoe. "Oh no! My Achilles has just gone again – taxi!"

Don't run after a heavy meal. Not all of us take the same amount of time to digest a meal or share the same tolerance to different foods.

Treadmills

The workouts I have prescribed in the following section can also be done on a treadmill, the choice is yours. I have divided the treadmill debate into 'for' and 'against'; in my opinion people either love them, loathe them, or will only use them if they can't get outside (I fall into this category). It must be said, however, they are immensely popular with gym users. Many runners get a decent level of fitness from them who would never set foot outside, for various valid reasons.

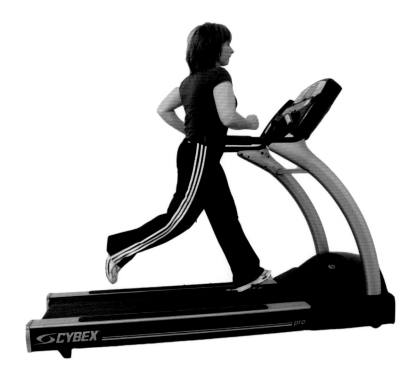

Getting going

LEVEL 1 and 2 (you will need a wristwatch)

1. Walk briskly for 5 minutes.

2. Pause for a short stretch (perform all stretches standing) and mobilise joints.

3. Note the time on your watch.

4. Jog for 5 minutes, turn around and jog back to the starting point, tapering off over the last few hundred yards, slowing to a walk.

5. Continue walking for 5 minutes to cool down, breathe deeply, take 5 deep inhalations through the nose as you walk.

6. Shake limbs out gently to loosen them. Stretch each body part for up to 30 seconds each. Try to do this lying down on a clean comfortable surface if possible. If you are going to stretch on your return home, enjoy a luxurious stretch on the carpet. It is wise to not only remove dirty shoes first, but also to check you do not have mud spattered up your back before going horizontal, as I have found this to be very poorly received.

Before the next stage

Check how you feel on the following two days. If you were sore and your legs ache, wait until the ill-effects have completely gone before setting out on your next jaunt. Old school runners may try to advise you that you can go straight out again and run it off – do not follow this advice, you will probably aggravate the situation and be laid-up for weeks. Instead – rest sensibly for a few days, which is usually all it takes. Likewise, never go running if you feel unwell. You'll most likely feel a sight worse after running; you need to be in good health for something as demanding as running – it is not for the sick.

If you felt fine afterwards, press on with (all in minutes):

Walk 5, run 10, walk 5, as before for another 4 weeks.

Once you can do this with some degree of comfort, step it up to:

Walk 5, short stretch, run 15, walk 5, long stretch (for another 4 weeks).

Then step it up to:

Walk 3, short stretch, run 20, walk 3, long stretch (for 6 weeks).

Doing this for three times a week will give you a decent standard of fitness. I must emphasise that if you have reached this stage and still find it challenging then you should stay with it until it becomes achievable without distress or major discomfort before considering taking the next distance on.

Three 20 minute runs a week for a person of 50-plus is an achievement if you have not run before or in living memory.

But, if you are ready to "kick on":

Walk 3, short stretch, run 30, walk 3-5 (according to how you feel), then have a long stretch.

If, up to this stage, you have been travelling at something between a plod and a lope, once the 30 minute run becomes routine, try to aim for a little more speed but only in short spells initially. See if you can cover more ground in your 30 minute run.

Fartlek (modified)

This excellent training system has not attained the popularity or respect that I feel it deserves but this is its own fault – it should have called itself something else; I pity any P.E. teacher trying to introduce it to youngsters. It is Swedish and means speed-play, which is how it should have been introduced to gain respectability.

It employs varied pace movement, involving running at different speeds interspersed with walking. It can be structured beforehand, so the runner sets out to cover pre-designed time periods at different speeds, or simply freestyle, where the runner pleases themselves whether they want to run, plod or walk. I prefer the latter, especially for beginners, as they can use this system to suit not only their level of fitness, but also their mood. Ideally it should be interspersed with continuous running – aim at a 30 minute target time but do not treat this time as if set in stone.

Once level 1 and 2 trainers have reached this level, and feel relatively comfortable covering 30 minutes of running (or jogging), move up to level 3.

Levels 3 and 4

If you are fit, but have never been involved in running, start out easy. If your fitness comes from other disciplines then running can make some demands on the unsuspecting.

Test the water with this simple 'taster':

Walk 5 minutes, take a short stretch, run in relaxed fashion for 10 minutes, walk 5 minutes, take a long stretch.

If this is easy (hopefully not insultingly easy though) then get ready to press on for some gainful progress. Step up your running time in 5 minute increments until you reach the 30 minute period.

You probably only need to walk briskly for 3 minutes before your short stretch. Do the same following your run, and take a long stretch. We are not all built or made the same way and some people, I have found, like a long-ish walk before and after running. Some never walk at all; you will have to find what suits you best. Once you develop the right formula for your running, use it as a base to increase your distance or speed, as you wish, to improve your residual fitness.

After this stage you may want to investigate running for longer distances. People over 50, men and women, who run marathons are a common occurrence these days.

Go-go girls - women lead the way

This report (from www.seniorjournal.com) did not amaze me, and will not surprise the frighteningly fit mature ladies out there - there are a lot more than most people realise.

According to a report by Peter Jowl M.D., a professor of orthopaedics at Yale School of Medicine, women lead the way in proving senior citizens show greater improvements in running times than younger runners. In studies taken of The New York Marathon from 1983-1999 they found women marathon runners aged 50-59 improved their average race times by 2.08 minutes every year, as opposed to their male counterparts, who only improved, on average, by 8 seconds a year.

The older males did, however, make greater improvements than younger male runners. Overall the greatest improvement in running times came in males aged 60-69 and 70-79, and women in the 50-59 and 60-69 age categories.

Fartlek

Ignore the clunky title; this is a brilliant training tool. Mix up your running, jogging, sprinting and walking over the duration of your workout. You can either structure your training beforehand, try it freestyle or experiment with which system suits your specific individual requirements. Continual change can help to keep your workout fresh and relieve any chance of boredom or stagnation.

There are more books written on running than just about any other sport, even golf and football. Some are instructional, others tell of personal case histories. The one I liked best, *Running and Racing Over 35* by Jeff Galloway, appears to be out of print. It helped me and several acquaintances train for a first-time marathon.

For and Against Treadmills

Fine when weather is snowy, stormy or otherwise foul.

If you feel a slight strain, you are not stranded miles from anywhere.

Recoverers from injury can give themselves a fitness check in a warm, safe environment.

Most modern treadmills monitor time, calories and pulse. They have miles or kilometres readouts to save mathematical gymnastics.

For beginners it can help to build confidence before "hitting the road."

Can be elevated for hill running. The lowest incline setting is suited to the faster runner right from the start of their run.

You can wear a walkman, discman, iPod or whatever in safety and, on most treadmills, store a drinks bottle easily to hand.

You have to stay on the pace, or finish up flying off the back (I have witnessed this twice; in both cases people did not operate the controls properly). Many models are compatible with heart rate monitors and help those training with them to stay in the required training zone. Not easy if you have to keep looking at your wrist receiver rather than up at the display screen in front of you.

There is no getting away from the unpleasant fact that some individuals sweat all over the treadmill and don't always mop up. If you have a tendency to perspire copiously, take a towel on board.

You will tend to run in a stride pattern that suits treadmill running. It will differ from your natural technique.

Other users get twitchy if there is a limited number of machines. Some clubs limit use to 20 minutes.

People have been known to make spectacular exits from treadmills, usually through looking at a TV monitor while increasing speed. I once saw a guy draped across a nearby pec-deck machine making this very manoeuvre. Treadmills must be treated with respect to ensure safety. Read any applicable safety warnings posted by the machine.

Some clubs, in the interests of safety, govern the speed quite drastically, inhibiting the faster runner.

Can get boring unless you have a TV or music to keep your mind occupied.

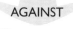

AGAINST

Other books worth a look at are:

Galloway J, "Running: Getting Started" (2005) Meyer & Meyer Sports Books

Whalley S, "Running Made Easy" (2004) Robson Books Ltd.

Burfoot A, "The 'Runner's World' Complete Book of Running For Beginners (2005) Rodale International Ltd.

Kowalchik C, "The Complete Book of Running for Women" (2000) Simon and Schuster.

Masters Athletics (monthly magazine). A magazine aimed directly at the older athlete and prospective older athletes. Full of sensible, hardheaded information from respected and revered experts. Gives details of upcoming events and results from past events. For those who are not already aware, the term *masters* (born in the USA) is fast replacing *seniors* or *veterans* in terms of older competitors.

18. Swimming for the Over-50's

My old friend Rob Springett, a full coach with the Amateur Swimming Association, currently coaching high-achieving juniors as well as his formidable and successful 'Masters' section at Chelmsford Swimming Club, supplies the following advice. I have never encountered a more enthusiastic or dedicated coach; he truely knows of which he speaks.

Swimming has long since been recognised as a fitness activity that you can do until you are ready for your box. Water is the medium of resistance and can therefore increase strength, endurance and flexibility. You can pull yourself through water as gently or forcefully as you desire, making this medium very flexible indeed, unlike the metal weights that you would use in the gym.

Cost

Most Councils will give concessions to us senior members of the public and therefore the cost is not prohibitive. If I were to generalise then I would assume that most of us could get a swim for between £1 and £3. Some pools have specific sessions for the over 50's and some even have ladies only sessions. This is fine as you begin your new fitness programme. After a few months you may feel the need to move away from these more sedate sessions and explore other pool times more appropriate to your needs.

Equipment

Equipment for swimming is also quite a bit cheaper than for most other activities.

To begin you will need a good fitting costume preferably with an endurance label produced by most well-known swimwear manufacturers. An endurance costume will last you quite a while longer than a standard one in the chlorinated water, provided that you rinse it well after use. Some of the newer swimming pools these days use very little chlorine as the cleansing or purification agent. Instead these pools use ultra violet lamps to kill bacteria, reducing the need for lots of chemicals and thereby reducing the wear and tear on our bodies and equipment. As well as a good costume you will need a kick-board, pull-buoy, fins and a good fitting pair of goggles. (Words highlighted are defined in the swimming glossary, page 135.) A drinks bottle is also essential. Once purchased, the costume and perhaps the goggles are all that will ever need replacing. A word of warning – never loan your goggles to anyone as it can take several sessions to get your goggles adjusted to suit your head and eyes and to obtain the correct pressure to prevent leakage.

Drinking

Drinking during your training session is very important. Swimming is no different to any other vigorous activity that you undertake, in as much as you will lose bodily fluids via perspiration. These fluids need to be replaced before you become dehydrated and thirsty. As a rule, if you exercise for about an hour you will need to drink a full litre bottle to maintain hydration. Don't allow yourself to become thirsty; always take sips little and often throughout your session. Your body will also need to have the glucose or sugars it uses up replaced, so I suggest that you do the following. Take your favourite fruit juice and dilute this by at least 50% of the total water in your bottle. To ensure that your body takes up the glucose as quickly as possible you will need to add an electrolyte. The most effective way of doing this is to add a quarter of a teaspoon of salt and shake well to dissolve. If you can taste the salt then you have added too much. The fancy – often very expensive – drinks that you can get from the reception and machines in the sports centre will sometimes do the job, but the much cheaper option is to make your own.

We have sorted out our equipment and know what sessions we are going to attend; we now need to go to the pool and begin our new fitness regime. At this point I can't emphasis enough that we have the rest of our lives to achieve our desired level of fitness. We do not need to be super fit by the end of the first week or month. If we accept that by doing any exercise we will be a little fitter at the end of the first week and even fitter after the first month, then we can enjoy the progress towards our eventual goal. Most of us who begin a swimming programme after the age of 50 have probably all swum at some level when we were younger. If however you are a non-swimmer, or still a learner, then I suggest that you contact your local council and speak to the Sports Development Officer. He or she will know if there are any adult "Learn to Swim" programmes in the area. These may be at your local sports centre or in local school pools.

How long do we need to swim when we are starting a new fitness programme? Let me start by saying that swimming equates to 4-5 times more than the equivalent of running or walking. That is to say that if you:

Swim 800 metres comfortably it is equal to 3500 metres walking.

Swim 1000 metres at 70%-80% it is equal to 4000-5000 metres jogging.

Swim 2000 metres hard effort it is equal to 8000-9000 metres running.

Apart from the beginner (or non-swimmer) there are three other levels of swimmer:

LEVEL 1 (Reasonably fit and healthy but not used to regular physical exercise)

I would suggest about twenty minutes maximum for the first couple of weeks. Most people in this group will swim using breaststroke only. Breaststroke coordinates the arms and the legs, whereas the other strokes coordinate the arms, legs and breathing. Most pools have a pace clock, which should be visible from either end of the pool. Swimming comfortably, you should swim between 20 and 30 lengths and time yourself for the distance. Much will depend on your initial levels of fitness and the overall time that you allow yourself for your visits to the pool. After a week or two of regular swims (once the aches and pains have disappeared) you will be able to judge how long it takes to swim, say, 30 lengths. As you get fitter the time will shorten quite considerably and now you will need to decide if you want to swim faster over the same distance, or increase the distance swum at the same pace. Either way you will increase your stamina and improve your cardiovascular system.

Level 2 (The fit over 50)

Several people are fit from their occupation or are very active in other ways. Some are LEVEL 1 swimmers who have progressed to this new level. These swimmers are now ready to structure a swimming programme to work different muscle groups and incorporate all of the energy systems.

Kickboards will isolate the front end (arms, shoulders, and torso) and encourage the swimmer to use the leg muscles. Pull-buoys are placed between the upper legs just below the crotch. This stops the swimmer from using their legs and so encourages the use of the core, chest and shoulders. Fins can be used to strengthen the legs whilst keeping the ankles both flexible and supple. Please note that some pools will not allow the use of fins. Apparently this is a health and safety issue, although I have never had a real explanation as to why it is dangerous.

Now that we have a structured swimming programme we must ensure that we allow enough time to warm up and swim down properly.

Level 3 (The very fit)

This group is mainly comprised of ex-competition swimmers, known as Masters. Competition swimmers and Masters squads are increasing in number annually.

Most leisure centres will have a swimming club associated within the complex and many of these clubs will have a Masters section. Masters training is the pinnacle of swimming training for the senior swimmer. Training with like-minded and similar ability athletes makes it much easier to motivate you to train harder and more regularly.

Before entering the water try to find five or ten minutes to do some stretching and flexibility exercises. Much of the activity in swimming is completed above the head. Therefore we must pay particular attention to shoulder flexibility. As well as good flexibility of the shoulders and ankles, we are often moving arms, legs and head together – this needs to be stabilised by using our core muscles. The core is our abdominal muscle group and other muscles in the torso. When using our arms, the primary muscle is the tricep and the stabiliser is the bicep. We also need to keep our wrists flexible for the various hand movements. Because we pull ourselves through the water from above the head – along the centre line of the body and finish at the hips – we bring into action the pectorals, the latissimus dorsi and the trapezius muscles. There are several smaller muscles that are essential to the swimmer but I think that we have enough to work on for now. If you have access to a good gymnasium and would like to improve your swimming then I would suggest the following:

1. Work on your core strength. This is now common practice in most gymnasiums and is excellent for general fitness.

2. Cardiovascular fitness. Try to spend about half an hour on bikes, treadmills, cross-trainers and rowing machines (altogether not each!).

3. In my opinion, avoid the free weights and stick to the machines. I always think that the machines are easier to control. There are several machines that will strengthen the muscles used when swimming: lat. pull downs, chest press, and tricep curls. Squat machines are also very good for our major leg muscles.

> **Tip**
>
> Please remember that swimming is a very low impact sport compared to working out in the gymnasium or jogging. If you have any injuries or mobility limitations then seek advice at the gym or just stick to gliding up and down the pool.

Some basic swimming programmes are shown below. These can (and should) be adjusted to suit the time that you have and your own desires.

Level 1 programme

Let us start by assuming that you are a swimmer who, a few years ago, could swim about 30 lengths (750 metres) breaststroke. Begin by doing 5-10 minutes stretching (in the changing rooms if you feel embarrassed to do it on the poolside).

You don't need any equipment for this first session. Take a note of the time, then begin by swimming for 5 minutes. Stop if necessary but try to keep the stops and their duration to a minimum. Count the lengths completed. Repeat this process (in 5 minute blocks) until you have completed 20 minutes of exercise. Make a note of the total lengths and your best 5 minute block. You can now have a shower and feel good about your first session. This is a very basic programme and should be repeated for about the first month.

In order to push yourself forward and increase your fitness and stamina:

Take an average of the number of lengths you can swim in a 5 minute block, (from a twenty minute session) and make that the minimum number of lengths you must now swim in 5 minutes. We will call this minimum length value z.

For the next block of programmes we need to begin using the pace clock. Commence the programme as usual by doing your stretching and 2 of your 5 minute swims, remembering not to go below z. You should now be fully warmed up and ready to increase your pulse rate. Check the pace clock and swim one length at approximately 80% to 90% effort (almost as fast as you can go) and note the time taken. Let us call this time y. We now add 20 seconds to y and this will give us our repeat times. Now see how many lengths you can swim trying to hold $y+20$ seconds.

For example if it took you 40 seconds to swim a length as fast as you can go (y), your repeat time would be 60 seconds. So now our programme is:

5 to 10 minutes stretching.

5 minute swim holding lengths at z or above.

8 times 1 length at repeat length time (i.e. y +20 seconds).

3 times 5 minute swims (holding z lengths).

This could be adjusted with regard to your time at the pool and fitness levels. The programmes above are designed to improve your aerobic fitness levels. It is possible to improve your aerobic fitness by just swimming as many lengths as you possibly can in a given time but I find this very boring.

When you have mastered these simple programmes and are very consistent with your times you may want to move on to an intermediate programme.

Levels 2 and 3 programme

You will require a kick-board for this session. You should now be able to swim for approximately 45 minutes with no breathing problems and no aches or pains from your swimming exertions.

Continue with your initial 5 to 10 minute stretches then do a warm up swim. Your warm up could be a *pyramid swim*. A pyramid is comprised of: swimming 1 length with a 10 second rest, then swimming 2 lengths with a 10 second rest, then swimming 3 lengths with a 10 second rest and then swimming 4 lengths with a 10 seconds rest. You then reverse the process from 4 lengths down to 1 length. Therefore, the programme would be:

- Swim a pyramid from 1 to 4 lengths on your favourite stroke (number 1 stroke), then swim 4 to 1 lengths with your second favourite stroke (number 2 stroke) (total distance = 500 metres).

- Swim 8 lengths of your number 1 stroke, aiming for y plus 15 seconds. Then do 4 lengths of relaxed swimming to recover. Repeat this combination twice. (Total distance = 600 metres.)

- Using a kickboard (holding it out in front of you) kick 6 lengths of breaststroke and rest for 15 seconds after every length. Count your number of kicks for the length and try to reduce the number every length by gliding after every kick. Try to kick more powerfully to improve technique and power. (Total distance = 150 metres.)

- Finish your programme by swimming comfortably 100 metres breaststroke; trying to increase your stroke length by gliding between every stroke. (Total distance = 1350 metres). Adjust each section according to your fitness levels and time at the pool.

Alternate level 2/3 programme

8 x 50 metres: swim 16 lengths front crawl or backstroke, with a 15-20 second rest every 2 lengths.

Start very slowly and try to swim each couple of lengths 1 or 2 seconds faster than the previous one. This is a very difficult exercise, so start very slowly for the first few (total = 400 metres).

Do 3 x 5 minute swims (holding z lengths) with 30 seconds rest between each 5 minute block (total = 600 metres).

Using a kickboard, kick 6 lengths, each length comprised of half a length front crawl and half breaststroke. Take 15-20 seconds rest between lengths (total = 150 metres).

Finish your programme by swimming 4 lengths, with 20 seconds rest between each one. Start fast and swim each length 3 seconds slower than the previous one (total 1250 metres for the whole programme.)

The more advanced senior swimmer will need to use all of the equipment that we described earlier. Here is a typical programme that a fit, ex-competitive swimmer might attempt (or when the LEVEL 2 programmes have become relatively easy).

Level 4 programme

Warm up with 32 lengths of front crawl, with twenty seconds rest between each length.

Every 8 lengths, increase your pace by 3-5 seconds (total = 800 metres)

In the main set 10 x 100 metres. No.1 stroke to No.2 stroke, swum off 1min. 45 seconds (total = 1000 metres).

Using fins, if the pool staff allow them to be used, swim 4 lengths on your front or back.

Swum off of 30 secs with 15 seconds rest every 4 lengths. Repeat 6 times (total = 600 metres).

Using a pull buoy between your thighs, swim 8 x 50 metres. Front crawl with a 15 sec rest (total = 400 metres).

10 x 1 length (own choice strokes) with 15 seconds rest. Decrease the pace every length (total = 250 metres).

Total session = 3050 metres.

Another programme for the senior, very proficient swimmer who prefers less front crawl :

Warm up with a pyramid, with lengths 1-5 as backstroke and lengths 5-1 as your own choice stroke, with a 10 second rest between sets.

Finish the warm up with 10 x 1 length front crawl off of 30 seconds, at an increasing pace (total = 1000 metres).

Main set: 8 x (2 lengths No.1 stroke + 1 length front crawl) swum off of 55 seconds + 30 seconds.

8 times: 2 lengths front crawl and 1 length number 1 stroke, swum off of 50 seconds + 30 seconds.

Total = 1200 metres.

Drills:

Using a pull buoy between your thighs, swim 8 x 3 lengths of front crawl off of 80 seconds. Keep the strokes as long as possible (total = 600 metres).

Swim down

Swim 8 x 1 length of the stroke of your choice off of a 15 second rest.

Each length should be 2 seconds slower than the previous one (total = 200 metres).

Total session = 3000 metres.

These programmes are just a few examples of how you can improve your fitness levels without the boredom of just looking at a blue line on the bottom of the pool. According to your capabilities you can pick-and-mix from any of the programmes to suit your needs or mood of the day. The times given are just very rough guides. In the beginning you may need considerably more rest between lengths or sets.

All of the sets in the programmes are aerobic, and are designed to get you fitter. You will of course get faster as you get fitter and improve upon your technique. The top end of the programmes are more accurate and these swimming times are much more realistic. If you work your aerobic energy system for approximately 30-40 minutes on a regular basis, maybe 3 or 4 times each week then you will become fitter. If you are concerned about your weight and waistline, a good aerobic workout can help to lose weight in conjunction with a good diet.

If you are able to swim the senior, advanced programmes that I have included in this chapter, you really should consider joining a Masters Swim Squad. Those of you who can't quite manage these programmes should also visit the Masters Clubs to see if you can fit in. A knowledgeable person who is ever ready to assist and offer advice nearly always coaches these squads. Costs are rarely prohibitive, and most Clubs do concessions for people out of work and pensioners.

When we seniors train we generally work the aerobic energy system. Most of our competitive years are behind us, and we just need to be aerobically fit, with the best condition pump (heart). The aerobic energy system is generally broken down into three categories: A1, A2, and A3.

A1 – the recovery process.

When we swim down after a race or hard training session we use this part of the aerobic energy system. Our body uses this system to get rid of any lactate that we have built up in the muscles. By using this energy system we can often prevent muscle soreness from occurring. To swim in this zone the athlete needs to swim at 50-70 beats below maximum heart rate. (I will explain how you take your pulse at the end of this section).

A2 – the maintenance process.

When we swim for a long session, reasonably hard, we are maintaining our aerobic fitness. There will be days when you do not want to charge up and down the pool, when you have other things on your mind. These are the days when you swim to maintain your levels, not to improve them. Swimming a session at 30-50 beats below maximum will ensure that your energy levels are maintained.

A3 – the high endurance process.

Swimming hard with short rest intervals will improve your aerobic capacity. It will improve your cardiovascular system and your volume of oxygen intake. A typical swimming set to achieve this would need to be swum at 20-30 beats below maximum to improve this system.

I would not suggest that you swim every session at A3 level. Like everything else that we do, to achieve the best results we need to do a little of everything. For example, if you swim 5 sessions in one week I would suggest that you do two A3 sessions, two A2 sessions, and an A1 session. If you swim at A3 pace every day then your body would get tolerant of this and eventually it will cease to have the desired effect.

All of the above pulse ranges are approximations. Generally the pulse ranges will work for most of us, but there are always exceptions. If you find it very difficult to achieve these tolerances then adjust down and enjoy your session.

To check your pulse, count the beats for six seconds, using the swimming pool pace clock. Put a zero on the end and this is your pulse. It's not an exact measurement, but it certainly gives us a good estimate. For example, 13 beats in six seconds, add a zero, and you have a pulse of 130 beats per minute. If you have a problem locating your pulse then try this:

Tip

Put your middle finger on your ear lobe. Run the finger down your neck, towards the shoulder. When you reach halfway, move the finger forward towards your wind pipe about an inch. You should now be able to get a strong pulse.

Don't spend too long looking for your pulse. Some of my swimmers spend so long trying to locate their pulse that when they do find it, they have recovered and the information is rendered useless. Just enjoy getting fit and staying that way. I have always maintained that when I die I'll be the fittest one down there!

A couple of good reference books to add to your library:

- *Swimming Coaching* by Joseph Dixon (1996). This is a very uncomplicated publication explaining the mechanics of all the swimming strokes in detail.
- *Swimming Drills for Every Stroke* by Ruben J. Guzman (1998). Another excellent publication with simple practices for every stroke.

Glossary of terms for swimming:

Pull Buoy: A piece of moulded polystyrene foam that is gripped between the thighs very close to the crotch. It gives buoyancy, whilst preventing the swimmer from using his legs.

Kick Board: A flat piece of shaped polystyrene approx. 18 inches long by 12 inches wide. It is held by both hands either side approx. half way along its length. It offers extra buoyancy whilst exercising only the legs.

Number 1 Stroke: This is either the best stroke or the favourite stroke of the swimmer. Number 2 Stroke would be the next best or second favourite stroke. Number 3 or 4 strokes would be the swimmer's worst or least favourite strokes.

Pace Clock: These are on the wall in most swimming pools and have a very large, visible sweeping second hand. The pace clock allows the swimmer to be accurate with rest periods or swim off times.

An example of a rest period swim is as follows: "Using 8 × 50 metres off a rest of 20 secs" means that after each 50 metres swum, the swimmer takes 20 secs rest. If the swimmer does the same set off of 1min 20 secs, then they start to swim every 1min 20 secs, regardless of how long they take to swim the 50 metres. For example, they may swim the first 50 metres in 1 min 5 secs, allowing 15 secs rest. The next 50 metres may take 1 min 10 secs, giving the swimmer just 10 secs rest.

19. Indoor Cycling (Static Exercise Bikes)

A stationary bike is probably the least expensive piece of fitness machinery you will be likely to require. The cheaper models have extremely simple designs, easily capable of home repair or adjustments should you be required to carry them out.

The only place I would locate an exercise bike is in front of a television set, preferably with a video or DVD player, failing this near a window that overlooks signs of activity. This diversionary device prevents me from losing the will to live; I cannot imagine many forms of exercise more mind-numbingly boring than sitting on a bike in the box room staring at the wall. Go into most major gyms and you will notice the machinery facing the TVs is invariably the bikes and elliptical trainers.

However, cycling does provide an excellent cardiovascular workout, whilst being easy on any creaky joints (unlike the pounding of jogging). Indoor

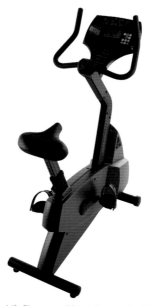

Life Fitness upright static exercise bike

machines provide everything outdoor cycling does – except fresh air and balance skills – and it is possible to work even harder on static bikes as many models allow you to elect to train on punishing, demanding courses for as long as you wish. It is also easier to reach for a sip of water, as even cheap models usually provide a handy holder and you can relax safe in the knowledge that you won't be needing to wear an unflattering helmet, be at the mercy of the weather or be bowled over by an articulated lorry.

There are quite a few considerations when buying an exercise bike and consequently some questions you should ask yourself:

All have display consoles these days but check it out before buying; do you need your glasses to read it? Does it make you squint because the display is so small or indistinct? If you don't want to exercise with your spectacles on get one with a large clear display console.

Weight tolerance: cheap models (e.g. Pro Fitness, £49.99 in Argos) have an upper weight limit of 16 stone. Life Fitness have a model at £995 with an upper weight limit of 28 stone.

Size: do you have adequate room? Upright cycles are not too demanding on space but recumbent cycles tend to be space hogs (apart from being more expensive).

Self assembly: does it come ready-assembled or do you have to get involved in DIY? How tricky is it to put together? The beauty of a second hand model is that somebody else has already assembled it.

How many facilities do you want the bike to provide? They all provide timers and miles per hour, distance covered and even the cheaper models usually give calories burned, although this last measurement is usually inaccurate. It is possible to get heart rate, pulse rate, calorific burn, wattage (I have never worked out how this could be useful), gel saddle (very practical in my opinion) and links to gaming systems or play stations. The Reebok Power Bike, amongst others, comes replete with an interactive games system to entertain you whilst pedalling.

Noise: air braking is where wind resistance is utilised by the provision of a big fan. One bonus is that it provides a refreshing blast of cold air up your heated legs (takes a bit of getting used to) but the noise level with most of these models is pretty high.

Those with back problems would be happier with a recumbent cycle which provides good lower back support. They are also easier to get on and off of, for people with physical difficulties, and gives a much more comfortable ride. If you feel wobbly when seated on an upright bike then this would be your best bet. The downside is that they can be fairly expensive.

Weight: how heavy is the machine? How strong is your floor when tested by a 16 stone man on a large recumbent cycle?

Cheapest models provide a range of preset programmes including: cardio, fat burn, target heart rate, hills, valleys and many more.

Quality of ride: this depends on the technical specifications and engineering standard, which will be reflected in the price. There are models driven by belts, which are the lowest priced; the belts provide a reasonable ride for the price when new but the fibres tend to wear away and you can finish up with drag, giving a jerky feel to the ride.

Another option is a steel flywheel bike – generally the bigger the flywheel the smoother the ride. The flywheel is controlled by magnets for braking, gives a smooth feel to the ride and makes less noise. The air-driven models are noisy but the Schwinn Airdyne, which has been going for as long as I can remember, is a good quality machine; it has no brakes as it uses wind resistance by virtue of a huge fan, and has a chain drive akin to a road bike.

Variations on the Bike Theme

'Dual Action' bikes

Dual action bikes use both arms and legs; cycles such as the Schwinn Airdyne require you to push the long ski-pole-like handlebars to and fro while you pedal, making this a much more demanding workout by involving muscles of the upper body (chest, back and shoulders).

Spinning Bikes

Spinning has become popular in the last few years and is usually performed in groups where an instructor calls the instructions out, whether it be sprints, hill climbs or other demanding routines. You need to be pretty fit to do these classes and I can only liken the saddle (you're up out of it half the time) like sitting on a large, dull knife. They are a good-looking piece of equipment, but whether you would get the use out of one at home is another matter entirely. This is one you should try before you buy.

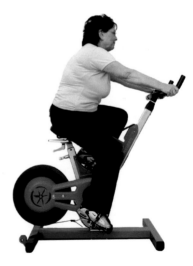

Keiser static Spinning bike

The X - Bike

A good-looking piece of quality engineering that simulates the feel of a mountain bike, and the handlebars torque from side to side, getting the upper body into the action. Not cheap but looks beautifully engineered.

Perhaps it's my age (my sons certainly think so) but I can remember when some of the prices for these things were what I would pay for a decent second-hand car, let alone any sort of bike, but if you have a bad back, desperately need to get fit and lose weight, three thousand pounds is merely relative to your needs. You could pay more in private health care and not feel any positive results; working out at least half an hour on a recumbent bike and your legs will let you know you have taken assured steps towards fitness.

> ## Tip
>
> Determine why you are buying an exercise bike. Everything hinges on your personal circumstances, be they physical or financial; I feel there is, in this competitive market, a bike at a reasonable price to suit your particular need, but take your time looking and you may just get a bargain.

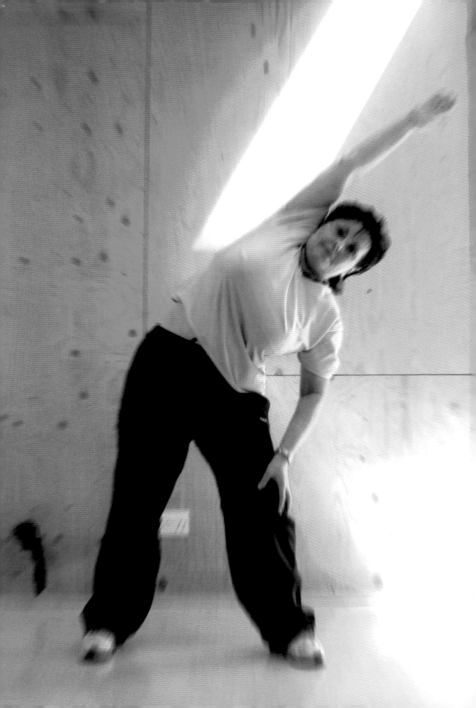

20. Cycling Outdoors

Whether indoors or outdoors, cycling gives a beneficial cardiovascular workout, targeting mainly the legs, buttocks and hip area.

The benefits of outdoor cycling:

Cycling works the heart with more intensity than walking.

Cycling does not involve the impacting or pounding of jogging.

Outdoor cycling takes away the tedium of static cycling and you get fresh, clean air into your lungs at the same time (although this obviously depends on where you cycle).

Reduces cholesterol and improves cardiovascular endurance.

Used instead of a car it helps reduce pollution.

Practical, as you can cycle just about anywhere, be it to work or for social visits or errands.

Cheap. Once you have bought your bike there is hardly any further cost other than minor maintenance.

The drawbacks are few but should be considered:

The possibility of injury. Riding a cycle through major cities carries an element of risk, mainly due to the indifference and lack of courtesy of motorist and cyclists who give the activity a bad name by riding on pavements, jumping traffic lights and failing to use lights after dark. City cyclists should always wear helmets.

Theft, again more prevalent in urban areas, but almost at epidemic levels in various larger cities. Thieves have become more and more proficient and bolder in devising ways to crack the toughest locking devices.

Getting involved in cycling clubs takes a good deal of overall improvement as they usually have a high standard of technique and endurance levels, making it daunting for mature newcomers.

Many urban areas suffer from a marked lack of dedicated cycle paths, making it hard for newcomers to gain confidence when forced to use roads with high levels of traffic.

To balance the pros and cons of cycling, The British Medical Association has estimated that the health benefits of cycling outweigh the risks by 20 to 1.

Making a Start

If you have had little to do with cycling but have decided this is the form of exercise you will most enjoy, start out by taking a 20-30 minute ride two or three times a week. At least you will find out this way if your backside and your saddle are compatible. Be advised by the store on saddle comfort and height of saddle to suit your needs. A specialised store will also be able to advise you on what sort of helmet you will need and other equipment, like shoes or gloves, you may feel you require. The average commuter cyclist should eventually aim for a fitness level that will enable him or her to complete somewhere between 2.5 and 6 hours a week.

Organised Cycling for the Seasoned Rider

The Cycle Touring Club is the UK's national cyclists' organisation with an estimated 70,000 membership. Apart from information on cycling, tours and events they provide insurance and cycling-related legal aid (www.ctc.org.uk).

I spoke to Mike Jackson, the secretary of the Chelmsford CTC, who informed me that although his group is referred to as the Over-40's club, the average age is nearer 50 to 60, ranging in age up to 80 years of age. Mike informed me the Attendance Winner – the member who turns out the most regularly on club days – was, in fact, a gentleman in his eighties. This form of club riding is not for the faint-hearted and anyone considering getting involved must be fairly experienced and durable, as the club members travel prodigious distances at respectable speeds. Routes are planned to use country lanes and spend as little time as possible on major routes. In the winter they will cover 50-60 miles a week but in the summer this is more likely to be 70-80, with two or three runs of over 100 miles. Preferred cycles are racers or touring bikes, some with twenty or more gears. It has to be said members are mostly people who have been cycling for many years, are returning to club cycling after a lay-off, or have switched from being proficient in activities such as running, but already have a good standard of residual fitness before taking up cycling as their major sport.

What Type of Cycle Do I Need?

You could go to a cycle superstore, or one of a chain of cycle shops but I feel if you go to a small specialised shop with staff that have been selling and maintaining bikes for years, you will get some sound advice from a knowledgeable specialist. Such a person is Mike Smith of The Cycle and Toy Centre (www.raleighinchelmsford. co.uk) and he offers this advice to the over-50's when looking for a suitable cycle:

"There are many makes, models and styles of cycles for all ages so choosing correctly is very important. First decide what sort of riding the cycle will be used for and shop wisely by going to a reputable dealer who sells quality brands and can advise you on your specific needs."

"The best style of cycle for the beginner, or someone getting back into cycling would be a hybrid. The hybrid is a cross between a racing bike, a conventional bike and a mountain bike, having features such as larger wheels like a racer, a more comfortable upright seating position like a conventional cycle, better gear ratios and often front suspension for more all-terrain cycling, like that of a mountain bike. These cycles start from as little as £170 for a fully aluminium bike. There is no need to spend more than £300 for a beginner or intermediate cyclist."

"For the more competitive cyclist such as a triathlete (swim, bike, run) or duathlete (bike and run) or anyone wanting to cover higher mileage in the shortest time, the best choice is a racer. This style of cycle is available with straight or drop handlebars and is for road use only. The riding position is more leant forward and aerodynamic for greater speed, and would not be the ideal cycle for a beginner as it is not the most comfortable riding position. These cycles start from a minimum of £300 to whatever you are willing to pay."

"There are other styles of cycles, such as the conventional 3 speed, which is designed for shorter distances (popping into town, or simply taking a leisurely bike ride for some fresh air and exercise). They are very durable as they are of a basic design, which means there is very little to go wrong."

"For the older cyclist who is still young at heart there is the mountain bike, which is an out and out fitness cycle, mainly for off-road use as the riding position is generally more bottom up and head down They are very low-geared for all terrain and the tyres are more knobbly and grippy for this use. The friction of the tyres on the road can cause a lot of drag and having 26" wheels makes for a much harder ride."

"The most taxing cycle to ride is the full suspension as this cycle has suspension on the front and rear and absorbs most of the rider's energy while pedalling. This style of cycle is purely intended for off-road and would not be recommended for any other use."

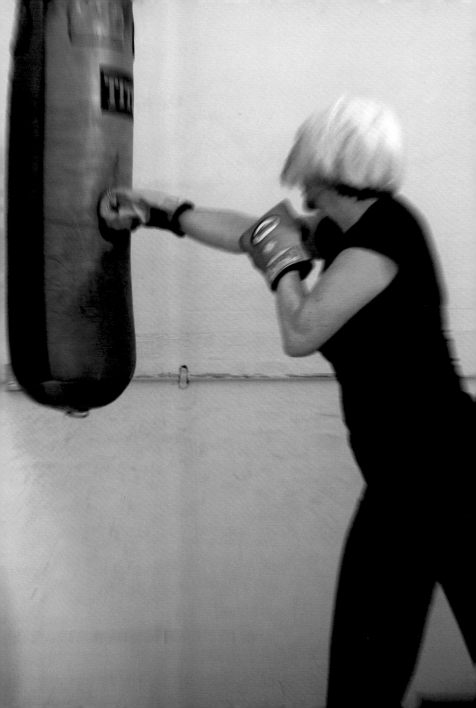

21. Rowing

Rowing machines are great for all-round fitness. They improve endurance and muscle tone even when working in a slow fluid movements. This is as good an indoor workout as you can get and proudly boasts to be a total conditioning exercise. It works great as a stand-alone exercise or combined with other activities. A good introduction is to use it as a warm-up before weights or an exercise class, and see if you like it.

Benefits

Improves aerobic activity.

Improves muscle tone; uses every major muscle group (Fluid Rower claim 84% of muscles used).

Improves stamina.

Weight bearing and impact free (no jarring of joints).

Ideal for older or heavier-built people.

Excellent for rehabilitation, especially those with knee problems.

Great as a component of cross-training, combining well with cycling and running.

Usually plentiful at most gyms (I have never seen a queue for the rowing machines).

Drawbacks

- Back sufferers should take professional advice to ensure the exercise does not aggravate an existing condition.

- Users need to develop correct technique to gain full benefit.

- The most common complaint is tedium, sliding to and fro for 20-30 minutes is not to everybody's liking; add some pretty hard effort to that and boredom can set in quickly.

Size

- The three major rowers are around 7-8 feet when extended, but the Fluid Rower and the Concept can be folded or stood on end.

Cost

Considering the standard of construction and quality, all three of the major brands (Concept 2, Water Rower and Fluid Rower) are competitively priced in the region of £800-£900, if they are to be used regularly – as they would make an expensive and space-hogging ornament/clothes horse.

Gym and home rowers

The best-selling rowers have differing resistance systems:

- Pistons: usually cheaper models use pistons and unfortunately they have a reputation for being fault-prone and have a poor 'feel'.

- Air: these rowers use a damper to vary resistance against fins rotating on a flywheel in a metal drum; they are generally very reliable.

- Water: these machines use paddles in a sealed drum filled with water.
- Electric/ magnetic/ friction: it is usually the budget models of rower that use this type of system; the action and reliability is often doubtful.

Before you buy one:

Measure the space intended (weight is irrelevant as the heaviest weigh under 11 stones).

Try one out at the local gym when they have a free open day, or go as a guest with a friend if you do not already belong to a gym.

Check out the after-sales reputation and warranty.

See if the instrumentation panel will give you what you are looking for. Get one you can see clearly, especially if you don't want to train wearing your spectacles. Instrumentation is important to 'log' your progress and get instant feedback.

Check how comfortable the seat feels. Picture how comfortable it will feel 20 or 30 minutes later. Does the sliding action feel smooth and reassuring? You do not want to spend your workout like a rider waiting for the bell at a rodeo.

Before you sit down:

Tie shoe laces and draw-strings on shorts or jogging bottoms securely. The only real risk in rowing is getting a dangling lace trapped in the sliding mechanism (a major embarrassment if occurring at the gym).

For the same reason tuck your t-shirt in to prevent it getting trapped under the seat.

Easy on the jewellery – rings can scrape against the handle or the adjoining finger, which can irritate or cause blisters. If your hands are getting roughed-up by wear and tear, try wearing weight-training gloves. Gloves designed specifically for rowing use are in the £15 locality, whereas weight training gloves range from about £4-£8.

Comfortable trainers are important, should be laced up properly and should always be worn.

After 30 minutes it is not unusual to get a little saddle-worn and get the feeling your backside has gone to sleep. If you know you have a tendency to suffer from this, it may suit you to provide additional padding. My favourite solution to this problem is to stop every 10 minutes (there is a 'rest' facility on Concept rowers) sip some water and stretch my 'glutes' before resuming my workout. This will have little, if any, detrimental bearing on your exercise.

If you think the boredom factor may be problematic, turn on the hi-fi or, after ensuring it is firmly attached, the iPod or walkman. I do this at the gym to shut out music other people may enjoy, but which reduces my will to live.

If you have never worked out on a rowing machine before it is wise to take it easy at first. Acquaint yourself with the effort, comfort and rhythm that will be required for a smooth workout, then have a few 5 minute tester sessions. As with other cardiovascular exercise, I recommend a short stretch beforehand and a longer stretch after your workout.

Technique

Having ensured you are seated comfortably, tighten the foot straps and before grasping the 'oar' (wooden or plastic handle) slide backwards and forwards a few times to confirm it feels fine. Remember – if it doesn't feel comfortable at this stage, it's not going to improve from here on in.

Resistance setting

On the side of the metal (or plastic) drum containing the fan is a lever calibrated from 1-10. Number 1 is the easiest and the higher you go the damper works to increase resistance.

Level 1	Start on level 1
Level 2	Start on level 2
Level 3	Start on level 4
Level 5	Start on level 5

It is not a case of the higher the setting the more you will derive from the workout. People intending to use a rower mainly for weight reduction should use a Heart Rate Monitor working between 60-70% and those employing RPE (5-6), and would be best suited to setting the resistance at 4 or 5.

1. The return position

In this you are comfortably seated with your hands hooked over the oar's rubber handles lightly but firmly, as opposed to grasping it in a tight clench. Your wrists should remain 'flat'. The chain is parallel to the floor – keep it that way in the stages to follow. Never let it elevate or dip.

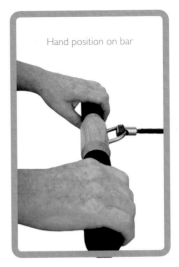

Hand position on bar

2. The 'catch' or beginning position

Keeping the chain parallel to the floor, move your upper body forward, bending at the knees so that your lower legs are vertical. Keep your head up and prepare to drive backwards.

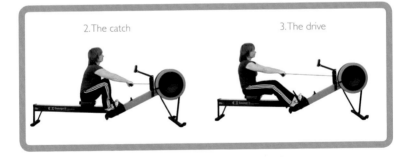

2. The catch

3. The drive

3. The drive

Pull the oar towards you as you slide backwards propelled by pushing through your legs. Keep your arms long until the oar passes over the knees. Make sure you keep your back straight and head up.

4. The finish

Your legs straighten out as the oar is pulled to the waist; your elbows should be drawn back past the body, with the lower arms parallel to the floor and wrists kept flat. Keep your head up and back erect, leaning back slightly on the conclusion, before returning to position 1, the return.

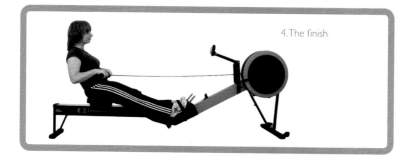

4. The finish

Do not:

   Whip the chain toward you – simply pull it toward you, evenly and smoothly

   Go off line – keep the chain parallel to floor

   Pull oar up to the chest – too high – pull to the waistline

   Raise the knees too early, forcing you to 'flip' the chain to clear them

   Use your back to achieve the drive – using your legs is vital

   Bend your wrists – keep them flat

   Twist the chain

- Forget to replace the oar in its holster

- Forget to adjust the resistance lever before getting seated, as you will have to undo the foot straps and dismount to do so.

Rowing Programme

- The first 2 sessions should be for 5 minutes at a rate of 25 strokes per minute.

- Then proceed to the next 5 minute increment once you feel comfortable and confident to make the step up.

- Levels 1 and 2 start at the very beginning.

- Levels 3 and 4 come in at 20 minutes at 28-30 rpm (if you have used a rowing machine previously).

- Row for 3 minutes at 25 spm; short stretch; row 10 minutes at 25 - 28 spm; long stretch.

- Row for 3 minutes at 25 spm; short stretch; row 15 minutes at 28-30 spm; long stretch.

- Row for 3 minutes at 25-28 spm; short stretch; row 20 minutes at 28-30 spm.

- Row for 5 minutes at 25-28 spm; short stretch; row 30 minutes at 30 -32 spm; long stretch.

Levels 1 and 2

Now try to increase the distance you cover, or the calories you burn in your workout. A 20 or 30 minute workout 3 times a week will keep you in good condition. Concept's website states:

> "The best guideline for weight-loss is to aim for rows of 30 minutes at a comfortably intense pace."

Level 3 and 4

Progress to a 45 minute session of varying speeds once a week

Try interval training of 3-5 minutes easy interspersed with 3-5 minutes fast.

Moving On

Concept's website gives a 'workout of the day', which is suitable for any rowing machine. It also has a training forum.

Group rowing classes, which are along the lines of cycle 'spinning' classes are gaining popularity at many gyms; an instructor calls the shots while everybody lines up on their rowers to toil at his commands. Worth trying once, I feel, but check with the instructor on the fitness level expected before diving in.

Rowing competitions are popular, with results published regularly in *Ultrafit Magazine*. Categories for seniors show the best times over various distances: 1,000, 2,000 metres etc. for the over 50's to the over 90's and they make impressive reading. These men and women are a testimony to the effectiveness of rowing as a physical activity that can keep you in peak condition.

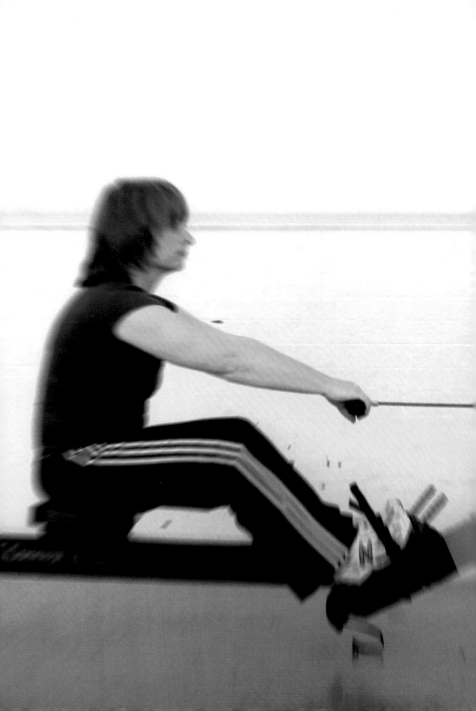

22. Elliptical Trainers

You may have seen these machines at gyms or health clubs and taken one look and thought to yourself *they look tricky* and to some extent they are at first. I would advise anybody over 50 who has never used an elliptical trainer to get an instructor to explain the technique and benefits before leaping aboard.

Most elliptical trainers employ magnetic braking to generate resistance, which can be varied greatly by the user, ranging from slow and steady to, frankly, hurtling – start with the former.

The machine has two long levers, which ape the action of the ski poles. They are driven to and fro in time with the leg action, which is an elongated circular movement that feels a little odd at first but soon becomes smoothly reassuring once you become accustomed to it. Like its outdoor counterpart it provides cardiovascular, endurance and strength benefits.

Hills and gradients can be simulated, as with the treadmill; the elliptical trainer burns a similar amount of calories, with less effort. The pounding of the treadmill is removed, making the elliptical trainer highly suitable for anybody with joint problems, especially dodgy knees. They are also user-friendly for anybody returning from injury.

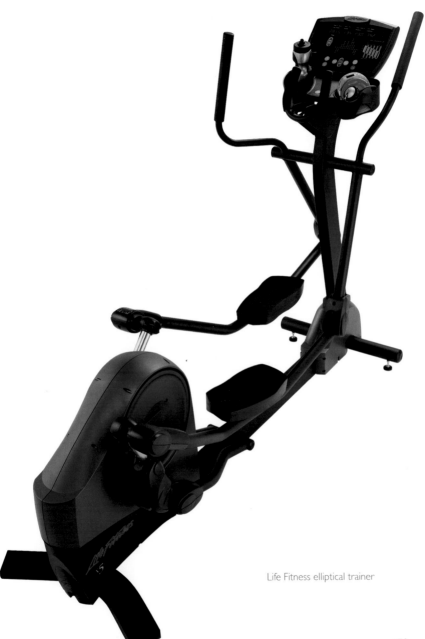

Life Fitness elliptical trainer

23. Skipping

If you are a newcomer to skipping or haven't tried it since your childhood, consider the following benefits:

1. Improves co-ordination; to skip effectively the upper and lower body must be in harmony and various muscle groups must work together to maintain your balance.

2. It allows aerobic training (will suit levels 1 & 2) and also anaerobic training, or a combination of both in a workout (will suit levels 3 & 4).

3. Increases joint strength and (as in most rebounding exercises) improves bone density.

4. Increases leg power and endurance.

5. Tones muscle and reduces fat.

6. Beneficial even when used in short periods of training.

Considerations

1. Length, material and quality of rope.

2. Surface to be used.

3. Footwear.

Ropes

There are numerous different types of rope but, for practical purposes I would recommend:

Levels 1 & 2: a simple leather or plastic 'rope'.

Levels 3 & 4: as above or a weighted rope comprised of plastic beads or tubing.

Level 4 could even try out ropes with weighted handles.

Length

All ropes need to be properly sized to suit the individual user according to height. A good test is to stand on the centre of the rope with the lead foot. The handles should reach the armpits. Taller people tend to be penalised in procuring a standard rope and often need to get one that is 'made-to-measure'. The rest of us can buy 'off-the-shelf'; the cheapest, reasonable quality rope I have seen was £2.99 but do not get a nylon cord, or fabric, as they lack the weight and substance to swing efficiently. You rarely need to pay more than £10 unless you want a specialist rope; you can get versions that will record the number of revolutions you make and the calories burned. A medium thickness leather rope with ball-bearings in the handles for a nice swivelling action will suit the beginner best of all.

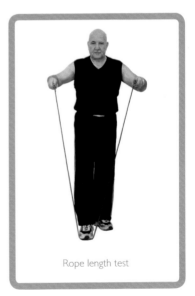

Rope length test

Level 3 & 4 only

Speed ropes (as the name implies) are fast-turning; made of slim but strong PVC and are modestly priced.

Heavy duty ropes are designed to strengthen the arms and upper body. Some have thick tubing for weight, others weighted handles for added resistance. Some versions combine both of these, are strictly for the determined trainer and only then in short bursts of 2-3 minutes to avoid excessive strain.

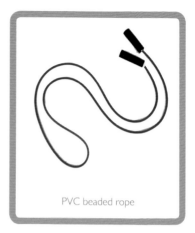

PVC beaded rope

Surface

Avoid concrete, tarmac or other equally unforgiving surfaces. The very least you will suffer is sore calf muscles. Ideally you need a sprung wooden floor or a rubberised gym floor. If you have floorboards or a laminated floor at home you just have to push back the furniture and heed the light fittings. Skipping on a carpeted floor is unlikely to prove harmful.

Footwear

Jogging or tennis shoes or cross-training shoes are all ideal. You need something fairly substantial to cushion your landing if the surface is a little on the firm side. Check your shoelaces are double-knotted as a loose lace will catch the rope and interrupt your routine. Bare feet are fine on a judo mat or a carpeted floor.

Other considerations

Long hair? Pin it down. Loose-fitting spectacles? Take them off or tie around back of your head.

Wear track trousers to begin with just in case you mistime a turn and give yourself a sharp slap across a bare calf muscle or thinly covered backside.

Ladies only – invest in a sports bra. You'll feel much better for it (so I'm informed). Spend a penny before you start (you'll have to trust my judgement on this one; I don't wish to go into pelvic floors and internal plumbing details at this juncture).

At this stage you may be saying, "Yes this is all very well for people with good balance and coordination but that's not me, I tend to be a little clumsy and uncoordinated. On top of that I'm not very fit."

To the first point I would answer: not to worry, skipping will teach you better coordination and improve your balance, which you may be glad of as you get along in years. You might not skip like Sugar Ray Robinson in all his pomp but you will be able to skip in some fashion if you follow the advice below and have patience.

Patience is an essential factor when first you attempt to skip. Using the technique I have outlined, some people I have taught have taken 20 seconds to skip, others (the minority I'm glad to say) may have taken 20 sessions before they felt a degree of satisfaction with their efforts. You do not have to look graceful or athletic, you just have to get a rope to pass over your head and under your feet – it's no more complicated than that.

Secondly, you do not have to be fit to learn to skip. Only somebody in pitiful condition would be too unfit to merely learn to skip. Regular skipping can then bring the reward of getting you fit, or at least fitter, according to the amount of time and effort you are prepared to invest in it.

Getting started

Where possible try to stand opposite a full-length mirror to monitor your alignment and to keep your head up; if you're looking in the mirror then you're not looking down at your feet, which will give you poor posture. To maintain a good ergonomic stance resist the temptation to keep looking down at your feet to see how they are doing! Stay tall at all times.

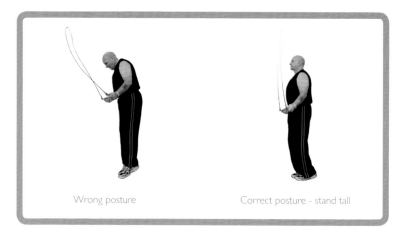

Wrong posture   Correct posture - stand tall

Get the rope to rest on the back of your knees, keep arms and legs loose and relaxed and start to bounce lightly on the balls of your feet with your feet about six inches apart – no rope yet! Once you established an easy, effortless bouncing rhythm that only takes you three to four inches off the floor, bring the rope over your head, clearing your feet with each revolution. You will hit your feet from time to time when you first start, which is frustrating just as you think you are mastering it. A good tip is that when this happens, don't stop bouncing. Just flip the rope over your head back to the start-up position, still maintaining your bouncing rhythm and then bring the rope back in again. This will help not only with your technique, it will save interrupting a continuous workout. It is purely a matter of timing the speed of the rope to miss your feet. It just seems more complex when you first start. Remember when you first learned to cycle, or drive a car? This is simple by comparison.

Once you have grasped the basics, improvement will only come by regular practice. Do not despair if success comes slowly, I have not had a single failure among the hundreds I have taught, no matter how uncoordinated or unfit they were. I am not going to pretend they all looked good – that takes time, effort and patience.

Get your breathing right. You may be surprised how tiring it is initially and if you are growing in confidence with your prowess, you do not want to then run out of gas. Breathe in quite deeply through your nose to maintain a regular breathing rhythm; don't hold your breath or become a 'mouth-breather.'

Bring your elbows gradually in towards your ribs and extend your thumb along the handle. After your first few minutes, if your calf muscle feels tight stop for a quick ten-second stretch; the calf muscles and Achilles tendon take a pounding when you skip (see section on Stretching, page 48).

For this reason I would advocate the perfect footwear for skipping to be running shoes with cushioned heels (with gel, waffles or air capsules in the heels) to minimise shock to the calf area (see Footwear, page 107).   .

Advisable timings

Level 1

Skip 2 minutes, rest 30 seconds. total start-up workouts 5 × 2 minute sessions

Level 2

Skip 3 minutes, rest 30 seconds; total start-up workouts 5 × 3 minute session

Level 3

Skip 3 minutes, rest 15 seconds; total start-up workouts 5-7 minute sessions

Level 4

Skip 3-5 minutes, rest 15 seconds; total start-up workouts 7-10 sessions

Cooldown / warm down stretch to follow – all levels.

Advanced techniques (but not too advanced)

Alternate Stepping

Start out in the two-footed bounce and then alternately place a foot in front, as if putting out a couple of cigarette butts! Vary this by taking a double beat with each foot.

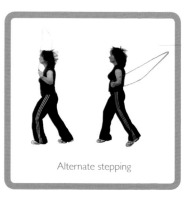

Alternate stepping

Ski Hops

Feet together, hop from side to side then switch to hopping backward and forward.

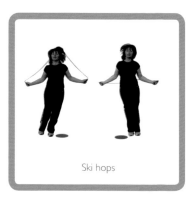

Ski hops

Split Steps

As you skip, start with feet together, then open to shoulder width and back again.

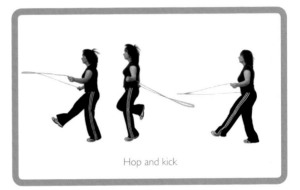

Split steps

Hop and Kick

Hop on one foot and take a small kick to the front – the classic-looking "boxer's skip."

Hop and kick

Leg Raise

Work the lower abs as you skip! While bouncing on one foot raise the other leg until it is bent at a right angle.

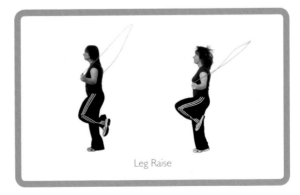

Leg Raise

Bumps

Finish a work-out off by jumping as the rope spins twice. See how many you can do, note it, then attempt to beat your own personal best.

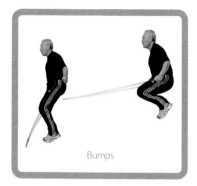

Bumps

Cross-overs

You will need a longish rope and the longer the handles all the better. Start off bouncing then cross your arms in front of you so the rope forms a loop, which you pass under your feet with a downward sweep of your crossed arms. Once the rope has flipped under your feet bring your arms back to the start position. At first it will take a little getting used to but think how impressive it will look once you can perform a continuous series of crossovers, a la Sugar Ray Leonard.

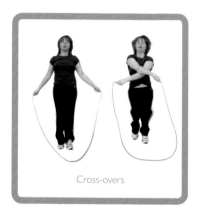

Cross-overs

Running in Place

Run on the spot as you skip, varying the pace but finishing on a flat-out burst. If you have a good space, jog forward and backward, or create your own variations on the running theme.

Back and Forth

Run forward for a few yards, then back up with alternating backwards steps. Alternatively, go forward and backwards with alternate steps, varying the speeds and stride patterns.

Skipping backwards

The ultimate skip challenge. Start with the rope resting on your shins and try skipping by taking the rope back over your head in the reverse direction. This takes quite a lot of getting used to!

Get Rhythm!

Dr. Costas Karageorghis, a sports psychologist, has confirmed what many of us already believed, that the right tune can help stimulate exercise. The secret, he believes, is in the type of music played; it has to be *synchronous* music, where the beat matches the body movement, rather than *background music*. His conclusion was that rock 'n' roll came out tops (*Unite Magazine*).

Skipping to music has a double advantage. It alleviates the inevitable boredom of skipping in silence, and is also helped by the tempo of the music. For people of a certain age, like myself, the perfect tempo record for beginners is Elvis Presley's 'Don't be Cruel', a steady repetitive beat lasting for only two minutes – perfect.

A repetitive beat works best to help you concentrate on your rhythm. Here are some others to consider, what I term *foreground music*, as opposed to background music. Some may, quite justifiably, curl their lip at my selection, but they have all been well tried and tested by friends. Judge for yourself.

My personal easy skipping top 20, in no particular order, is:

Don't be Cruel - Elvis Presley (2 minutes).

California Girls - Beach Boys (2 minutes and 30 seconds)

The Tide is High - Blondie (4 minutes and 30 seconds)

Green Onions - Booker T & the MG's (2 minutes 50 seconds)

Reelin' in the Years - Steely Dan (4 minutes 25 seconds)

Summertime Blues - Eddie Cochran (1 minute 55 seconds)

I Can't Help Myself - The Four Tops (2 minutes 40 seconds)

Ain't Got No - I Got Life - Nina Simone (2 minutes 10 seconds)

Take it Easy - The Eagles (3 minutes 30 seconds)

The Fat Man - Fats Domino (2 minutes 40 seconds)

Satisfaction - Rolling Stones (3 minutes 40 seconds)

Get Back - The Beatles (3 minutes)

Down on the Corner - Credence Clearwater Revival (2 minutes 45 seconds)

What a Fool Believes - The Doobie Brothers (3 minutes 30 seconds)

Dancing in the Dark - Bruce Springsteen (4 minutes)

There She Goes - The La's (2 minutes 40 seconds)

Let's Go - The Cars (3 minutes 30 seconds)

Night Train - James Brown (3 minutes 25 seconds)

Blue Suede Shoes - Carl Perkins (2 minutes 12 seconds)

1, 2, 3 - Len Barry (2 minutes 20 seconds)

Night Train was former world heavyweight champion Sonny Liston's favourite, which he would skip to at exhibitions. The somewhat hackneyed *Eye of the Tiger* (3 minutes 40 seconds) tends to go down well at our gym, but you will be able to find your own favourite once you try skipping to it.

Apologies for my choice being mainly set in the last century, but in a book on fitness for the over fifties I can't see The Prodigy or Eminem catching fire, or your CD collection containing 50 Cent or The Nine Inch Nails. However, many newer artists produce great music to use for skipping (including U2, The Red Hot Chilli Peppers, Oasis, Moby and many others) so why not borrow your offspring's CDs and experiment. Opt for something motivational, inspirational and uplifting, so, although I like them both in their way, leave Richard Wagner and Leonard Cohen in the rack.

24. Circuit Training At Home/ At The Gym

With and Without Equipment

You may have done circuit training before, possibly at a gym or as part of training for football, rugby or similar sports, that require a combination of strength and stamina. It usually consists of a number of exercise *stations* set around a hall or gym space, which you work out at for either the allotted time or number of repetitions and then progress onto the next station. Doing it at home will be slightly different (unless you inhabit a cavernous mansion or loft) but for those training in the box room, shed, garage or wherever you have chosen, you will be doing it in the confines of that space, merely picking up or putting down different exercise apparatus. It is not complicated, I assure you.

The beauty of circuit training is its flexibility to be adapted to specific forms for individual fitness or training needs.

Unless you are doing the class at a fitness centre and somebody is keeping the tempo by barking out instructions, you can feel free to go at your own pace; I would suggest working 30-40 seconds at each station. The type of circuit I have provided in this section is purely an example; you can modify it to suit your personal aims. I always try to spread out the pushing and pulling exercises so they never run consecutively; the biceps (used in pulling) and the triceps (used in pushing) are among the smaller muscle groups and need longer to recover. I also spread out the leg exercises as I feel it may prove debilitating to perform them consecutively in a circuit, unless a weight-bearing exercise such as squats is followed by an aerobic exercise such as skipping or jogging.

Decide if you want to focus on aerobic fitness, muscular strength, endurance or, as I favour in my examples, a combination of each.

The 'No Kit' Circuit

For the benefit of those who have yet to accumulate training equipment paraphernalia, I have devised a circuit that you can do at home without any equipment other than a solidly-built chair or bench seat.

Levels 1 and 2

Rest only a maximum of 30 seconds between stations.

Level 3

Rest 20-30 seconds, according to intensity.

Level 4

10-15 seconds, according to intensity.

> ## Tip
> Keep water handy – sip as you go. This is crucial in order to keep your heart rate up as you move through the circuit (see over the page).

Warm-up: 5 minutes of jogging in place, skipping or shadow boxing (see Boxing Training, page 192).

Mobility exercises (see Mobility, page 95)

Short stretch (see Stretching, page 48)

1. Press-ups

Level 1: box press-ups (performed with knees on mat) 10 reps.

Level 2: box press-ups (performed with knees on mat) 20 reps.

Level 3: 10-15 full press-ups.

Level 4: 20 press-ups, or 30 seconds continuous.

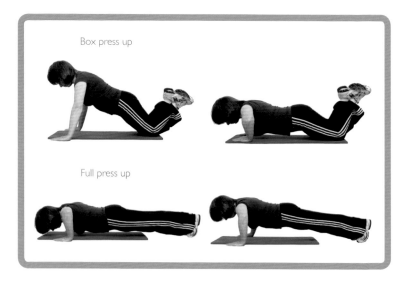

Box press up

Full press up

2. Step-ups (use stairs or doorstep)

Level 1: 10 step-ups each leg

Level 2: 15 step-ups each leg

Level 3 & 4: 20 step-ups each leg

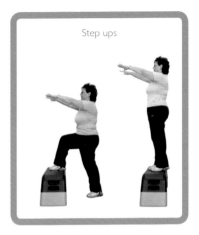

Step ups

3. Back extensions

Level 1: 10 reps

Level 2: 15 reps

Level 3 & 4: 30 seconds continuous

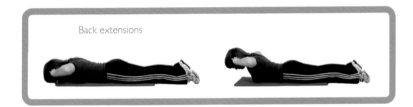

Back extensions

4. Shadow box

Level 1 & 2: 30 seconds relaxed

Level 2: 30 seconds – fast

Level 4: tuck jumps 20-30 seconds

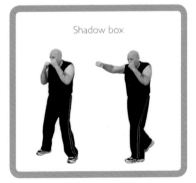

Shadow box

5. Curl-ups - abdominals

    Level 1: 10-15 curl-ups

    Level 2: 15-20 curl-ups

    Levels 3 & 4: crunches for 30 seconds continuous

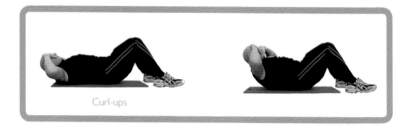

Curl-ups

6. Stick hops (any stick will do!)

    Level 1: 12 hops

    Level 2: 20 hops

    Levels 3 & 4: 30 seconds continuous

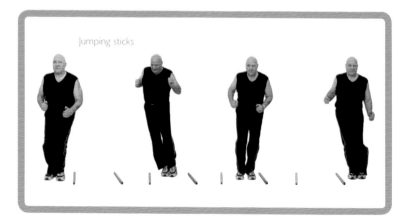

Jumping sticks

7. Calf raises

Level 1: 10 reps (from flat surface while supporting upper body)

Level 2: 20 reps (from flat surface while supporting upper body)

Level 3 & 4: 30 seconds (on stairs or step, supporting upper body)

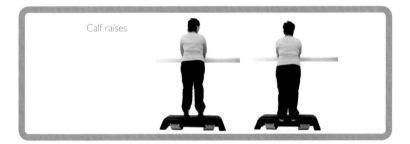

Calf raises

8. Chair dips

Level 1: 10 reps

Level 2: 20 reps

Level 3: 30 seconds continuous

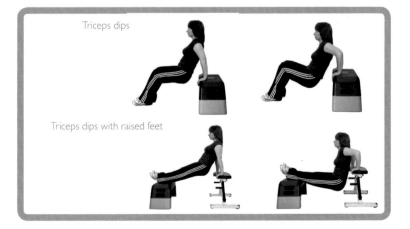

Triceps dips

Triceps dips with raised feet

Level 4: as above with feet elevated on another chair or box

9. Jumping jacks

Level 1: 10-15 reps

Level 2: 15-20 reps

Levels 3 & 4: 30 seconds continuous

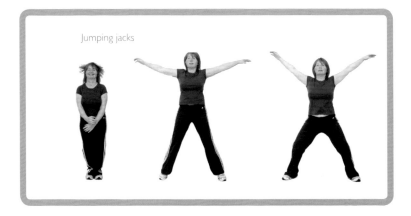

Jumping jacks

10. Squats

Level 1: 10 reps

Level 2: 15 reps

Levels 3 & 4: 30 secs continuous

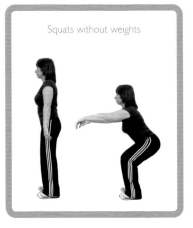

Squats without weights

11. Reverse curls

Level 1: 10 reps

Level 2: 15 reps

Level 3 & 4: 30 secs continuous

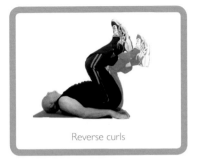

Reverse curls

2. Lunges/ high knee lifts

Level 1: knee lifts (so upper leg is parallel to floor) 10 reps each leg

Level 2: knee lifts 30 seconds continuous

Level 3 & 4: alternate leg lunges 30 seconds continuous

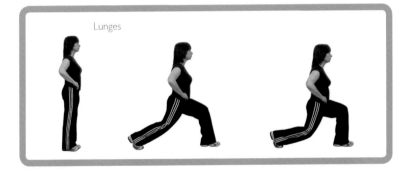

Lunges

13. Squat thrusts/ burpees

Level 1: 10 reps

Level 2: 15 reps

Level 3: 30 seconds continuous

Level 4: burpees – 30 seconds continuous.

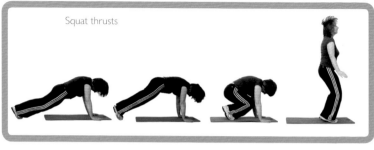

Squat thrusts

14. Plank

Level 1: 20 seconds (on knees)

Level 2: 30 seconds (on knees)

Level 3 & 4: 'full' plank 30 seconds

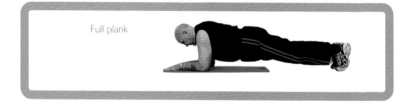

Full plank

15. Dorsal raise (lifting alternate leg & arm simultaneously)

Level 1: 20 seconds

Level 2, 3 & 4: 30 seconds

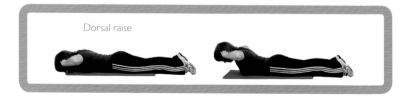

Dorsal raise

Warmdown: 5 minutes of relaxed skipping, shadow boxing or a 5 minute walk. Warmdown stretch.

To move on from this stage you can gradually incorporate some home-friendly, equipment – it can live in the garage, shed, loft or even the cupboard under the stairs if you can squeeze it in.

Equipment for Circuit Training at Home

Fit-Ball/ Swiss Ball/ Exercise Ball

A Fit-ball, Swiss Ball, Exercise Ball or whatever you want to call it (it's just the *big ball* at our gym) is great for both versatility and fitness improvement – improving your balance as you age is a boon as falls can be a grave problem in the later years. For an in-depth look at training with this apparatus, see the section on Core Training (page 56).

Skipping Rope

Skipping can be done at whatever pace you like – you will still derive some benefit from it. Ropes are cheap (I've seen them for as little as £2.99) but spending about £10 will get you a top quality specimen. For all you ever needed to know about skipping and skipping ropes see the Skipping section (page 160).

Tubi-Grip/ Exercise Tubing

Tubi-grip (also referred to as Exertube) is another useful addition, allowing you to do resistance training without using weights; it is versatile and reasonably inexpensive. It is colour-coded to reveal the degree of difficulty, black being the most resistant; green tubi-grip is ideal for those at Level 1. Reebok market a variety that is adjustable in length and comes in four varying strength levels.

Dynabands/ Exercise Bands

These stretchy latex strips, usually three feet by six inches in size (but can be bought by the roll and cut to required length) are a simple but effective training tool, allowing the user to perform a wide range of pushing and pulling exercises. The main problem as I see it is that there is no universal colour code; suppliers use their own colours for differing strengths, which can be confusing. Dynabands, a brand name that I (and most fitness instructors in the U.K) would recognise, use a colour code as follows:

Beginner = pink

Intermediate = green

Advanced = black

A colleague, Personal Trainer and fitness professional, Samantha Russell, advocates the use of bands for the senior trainer, or newcomers to exercise, who can start off with the easiest band, making them more user-friendly than some other forms of apparatus, which can appear more daunting.

Another virtue is that as they are small and light you can take them with you wherever you go – they can fit in your pocket or handbag. Training at home with them can be combined with other items, such as the Fit-ball, or just wrapped around a stair post to give an improvised pushing or pulling station.

I would advise buying two bands initially, one for exercises that use lighter resistance (e.g. tricep kick-back) and another for heavier work (e.g. seated rows) (see Bands and Tubes Workout).

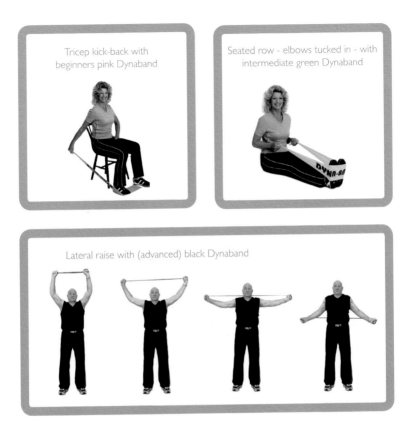

Tricep kick-back with beginners pink Dynaband

Seated row - elbows tucked in - with intermediate green Dynaband

Lateral raise with (advanced) black Dynaband

Weights

I have discussed weight training equipment in 'Free Weights Home Workout' (page 230) but I feel I should emphasise that a set of different weights will be of great value for home circuit training, as you will have more variety. The weights you perform squats with will, ideally, be a little heavier than those you do lateral raise or bicep curls with, but only buy what you need, especially if you are only going to use them once or twice a week.

Stepbox

Reebok (as well as other brands) market a purpose-built step box/ Alternatively, get hold of a sturdy milk/bread/packing crate or use your (or a friend's) woodworking skills to assemble your own box.

People under 10 stone (63.5 kg / 140 lb) could use a strong, non-slip plastic step unit of the type sold in household stores, intended for shorter people to reach high shelves. I would not recommend anybody heavier than 10 stone or with foot size larger than an 8 or 41, for safety reasons. Place a rubber mat underneath it for added stability.

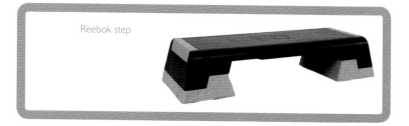

Reebok step

Punch bag

As discussed in detail in 'Boxing Training' (page 192), a punch bag is the greatest stress reliever I know of. Berating a punch bag for a few minutes allows feelings of tension and anxiety to ebb away from you, starting at about £30 (vinyl/PVC). Brands such as BBE, Blitz or Tornado all do a good line in affordable boxing equipment. A high-end leather bag by Reyes or Everlast will take you into the three figure bracket, but again you get pretty much what you pay for in this market.

Utility Weights Bench

A purpose built bench can be bought new for around £60, the Reebok bench at Argos can be used in a flat position for exercises such as *bench presses*, or as a seating unit for exercises such as the *seated shoulder press*. Benches can be quite easily picked up second-hand, and even a solid bench with a worn or tatty-looking cover can be re-covered quite simply and cheaply.

The Reebok Deck

I feel it is worth making a brief mention of this piece of equipment. It can be used as a step-box, a higher platform box, or a weight training bench (as long as you are not incredibly tall or over 20 stone). It also can be used as an incline bench and a decline bench. It has a compartment for rubber exercise tubes, which can be slotted into recesses in the bench to enable them to be used for resistance. I have no affiliation to Reebok but have to admire the designer who came up with this versatile piece of apparatus, which is perfect for using in the home circuit. It also comfortably passes my 'sturdy' test. The sting in the tail is that it costs £85 at time of writing, although I don't think that is too outrageous, unlike some other products I could mention, which I feel are monstrously overpriced.

Rebounders/ Trampette

Bouncing on one of these mini-trampolines puts little stress on the knees and can assist in improving your balance. You need to pick up a little speed to raise your body temperature as, given the nature of the apparatus, it does a lot of the work for you. You can make it a little harder by holding small hand weights. Two considerations are: is it sturdy enough to take my weight (some state an upper weight limit) and where am I going to store it?

Exercise Mats

Vital! You absolutely need one of these. Even if you have a luxurious carpet in the lounge or bedroom, you should still get a mat, in order to train comfortably anywhere you like. No need to pay the earth, I have seen versions that sell for £1.99. However, if you suffer from back problems it might be worth paying a bit more for a mat with thicker padding for extra support.

Home Circuit Workout with Equipment

	Warm-up: skipping, cycling or take a jog	5 minutes
	Mobility: as before	
	Short stretch: as before	
	N.B. Only rest a maximum of 30 seconds between stations	
1.	Press-ups	
	Level 1: box press-ups	10 reps
	Level 2: box press-ups	20 reps
	Level 3: full press-ups	10-15 reps
	Level 4: full press-ups or 30 seconds continuous (level 4 can increase degree of difficulty – see 'press-ups')	20 reps or 30 secs continuous
2.	Step-ups	
	Level 1: step-ups	10 reps each leg
	Level 2: step-ups with light weights	10 reps each leg
	Level 3: step-ups with moderate weights	30 seconds continuous
	Level 4: step-ups	30 seconds with (tolerably) heavy weights
3.	Back extensions	
	Level 1: back extensions	10 reps
	Level 2: back extensions	15 reps
	Levels 3 & 4: back extensions on Fit-ball if possible	30 seconds continuous
4.	Abdominals: reverse curls	
	Level 1	10 reps
	Level 2	15 reps
	Levels 3 & 4	30 seconds continuous
5.	Skipping	
	Level 1 & 2: gentle / easy skipping	30 seconds

	Level 3: fast skipping	30 seconds
	Level 4: flat out	30 seconds
6.	Shoulder dumbbell press	
	Level 1: using light weights	using light weights
	Level 2: using light weights	15 reps
	Levels 3 & 4: using moderate weights	30 seconds continuous
7.	Bicep dumbbell curls	
	Level 1: using light weight or tubi grip/ Dynaband	10 reps
	Level 2: using light weights	15 reps
	Levels 3 & 4: using moderate weights	30 seconds continuous
8.	Tricep dips or dumbbell extensions	
	Level 1: tricep dips	10 reps
	Level 2: tricep dips	20 reps
	Level 3: dumbbell extensions using light weight	15 reps
	Level 4: dumbbell extensions using moderate weight	20 reps
9.	Abdominals - curl-ups	
	Level 1: curls on Fit-ball or floor	10-15 reps
	Level 2: curls on Fit-ball or floor	15-20 reps
	Level 3: curl-ups on Fit-ball or floor	30 seconds continuous
	Level 4: curl-ups on Fit-ball holding light weight or medicine ball	30 seconds continuous
10.	Lateral raise	
	Level 1: lateral raise with light weights or tube grip/ Dynabands	10 reps
	Level 2: lateral raise with light weights or tube grip/ Dynabands	15 reps
	Level 3: lateral raise with light weights on Fit-ball	15 reps
	Level 4: lateral raise with moderate weights seated on Fit-ball	20 reps

11.	Squats	
	Level 1: squats with light weights	10 reps
	Level 2: squats with moderate weights	15 reps
	Level 3: squats with moderate weights	20 reps
	Level 4: squats with heavy weights	20 reps
12.	Single arm rows	
	Level 1: rows with light weights	6 reps each arm
	Level 2: rows with light weights	10 reps each arm
	Level 3: rows with moderate weights	10 reps each arm
	Level 4: rows with heavy weights	10 reps each arm
13.	Calf raises (two legs simultaneously)	
	Level 1: calf raises with a light weight in one hand - supporting upper body with upper hand (from flat surface)	10 reps
	Level 2: (performed as above)	15 reps
	Levels 3 & 4: calf raises holding moderate weight (using step box for maximum up and down movement)	30 seconds continuous
14.	Twists (remember to only turn 90 degrees - no full rotation)	
	Level 1: twists holding medicine ball/light weight	10 reps each side
	Level 2: twists holding medicine ball	12 reps each side
	Level 3: twists holding medicine ball	15 reps each side
	Level 4 'Russian Twists'	30 seconds continuous (or 15 reps if no Fit-Ball)
15.	Plank	
	Level 1: half plank on knees	20 seconds
	Level 2: half plank on knees	30 seconds
	Levels 3 & 4: full plank	30 seconds
	Cool down: skipping or jogging	5 minutes
	Cool down: stretches as before	

Taking it to the Gym

The workout shown above can be done at the gym should you prefer; their weights and facilities are probably vastly superior to anything you have at home, as your house is your home, not somewhere dedicated to training. The gym probably runs circuit training based on resistance training. Try a class - if it is not to your liking then do your own thing. The beauty of the class is that the instructor guides you with technique and what comes next; conversely, if you work alone you can go at your own pace and install your own variations.

In the weight training section there is a section on using gym machines for your circuit.

Where to find them/ how to do them:

1. Press-ups: page 74, 174

2. Step-ups: page 82, 175

3. Back extensions: pages 85, 175

4. Reverse curls: page 62

5. Skipping: page 160

6. Shoulder press: page 232

7. Dumbbell curls: page 234

8. Tricep dumbbell press: page 235

Tricep dips: pages 87, 177

9. Curl ups: page 59

10. Lateral raises: pages 233

11. Squats with weights: page 234; Squats without weights: page 82

12. Single arm rows: page 232

13. Calf raise: page 83

14. Twists: page 66

15. Plank: page 64

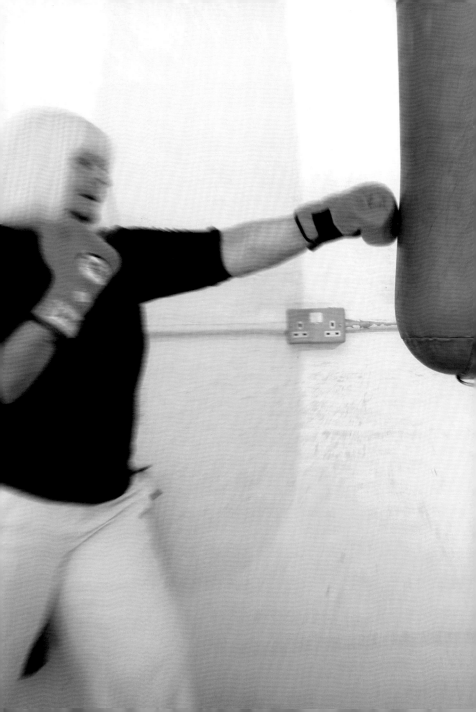

25. The Boxing Workout

If you have grown tired of all the other training regimes you have tried, why not give the boxing workout a go? You may find it refreshing; I tried it out on the folks in this book, Sally, Doug and Alex, and all of them agreed it made a nice change from the other elements of physical activity they had tried. It is akin to circuit training but using boxing associated exercises.

Why Boxing Training?

It improves strength, speed, coordination, agility, aerobic and anaerobic fitness and muscular and cardiovascular endurance.

If you are suffering from feelings of frustration or anger, I can assure you that bashing a punch bag will give you a refreshing sense of release, and make you feel a whole lot better. A middle-aged, physically disabled lady would come to our gym for about 20 minutes in the quiet of the afternoon and pound the heavy bag in 16 oz. gloves. She would leave in a calm, serene mood, telling us how much better she felt. She only needed the most basic instruction, "I only want to know how to hit it hard, dear," was her request. The same goes for you, so, if you have never hit a bag before, I will try to explain the best and safest technique for getting the most out of it.

The Where and the When

If I ever clear the junk from my garage I could hang my punch bag back up, make a space to skip and stretch, do my step-ups on my milk crate and do my shuttle runs by running up the road. If I couldn't get to the gym I would have to hire a skip to clear the junk out — as boxing training (or any form of martial arts training for that matter) is my favourite form of exercise.

If you do not have any home space for this workout you need to seek out an appropriate gym. It may be one of those new, air-conditioned, shiny gyms with racks of equipment but it may well be a converted church hall, with a wooden floor and fluorescent lighting; it may well be more gritty than glamorous. Even the new gyms have realised that there is more to boxing fitness than they previously considered and have installed punch bags and employed instructors who will teach people to skip rope, hold focus pads and teach people how to box. Ideally, you need somewhere that has access to a punch bag and space to skip and do your shuttle runs; many gyms have a quiet time between the lunchtime and evening class (I know our gym does) when you can take advantage of such facilities.

Equipment

It is possible the gym is where you will find your punch bag but if you have to get one at home the range is quite wide; ranging from £30 for the vinyl variety, or the costly but top quality Everlast or Mexican Reyes makes. For about £90 you can buy a decent leather (filled) bag; it is wise to buy a filled bag. Home filling never comes up as well as the manufacturer's product.

If you are buying for the home make sure you have somewhere strong enough to suspend your bag from.

Main Considerations for Home Use:

Structural damage

People often fail to recognize the stress engendered by continual sessions on even a light bag. Bringing the ceiling down can prove more costly than gym membership; a risky venture in the average home. If you are tempted to install one, ensure you consult a trusted architect or builder first.

Noise

Your neighbours are likely to suffer if there is a constant tattoo and dull thuds rendered by your efforts.

Fittings and fixings

These can be costly if you have to employ somebody to install it and (unless space is not at a premium) you will have a storage problem. Your nearest and dearest might not consider a punch bag an attractive feature if constantly on view.

The answer may be a free-standing bag, which range from £130-£250. Unlike a bag that hangs from the wall they allow for 360 degree movement.

If you are hanging the bag at home you will need a hook or a bracket (around £20 to £45) and a chains set (starting at around £7).

Gold's Gym retail a free-standing combined 'boxing stand', punch bag and speedball for £165, but with a base of over 4' it will need a generous space and a solid structure to house it.

There are different variations of punch bags; if your gym has a teardrop bag, an uppercut bag or similar then why not try them out. If you are a newcomer and the heavy bag is a little unforgiving try starting on something less demanding.

Hands and Gloves

I always advise getting your own gloves. If you have delicate hands you should wear sparring gloves, which are larger and more heavily padded to protect your hands. Otherwise, you will need bag mitts.

Always go for good quality leather mitts; the vinyl type tend to wear quickly, offer less protection and split easily. Make sure you have a little room in your new gloves, for two reasons:

Your hands will become hot if you wear the gloves for a long session and they will expand. Snug-fitting gloves will prove uncomfortable.

You will possibly want to wrap your hands, especially if you work on the heavy bag. Leave enough room for the wraps.

Hand wraps

There are readymade wraps, which you can wear inside your mitts, but I prefer the elasticated variety that you wrap yourself, as they can be formed into a perfect fit and are less likely to become unraveled with use. These have a Velcro fastening; the ones that need tying require outside help. Your wraps will lessen any abrasive rubbing from the glove and assist in keeping a straight wrist, in line with the knuckles and not 'cocked', which causes wrist injury.

Footwear

As the workout involves skipping and shuttle runs I would advise wearing running shoes.

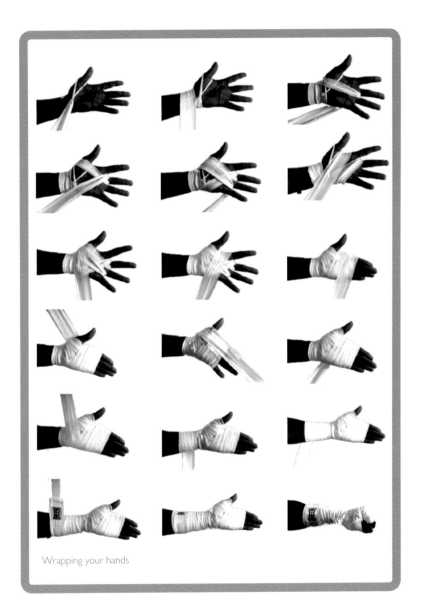

Wrapping your hands

Get the Most out of a Boxing Workout —————

The information I give here is for right-handed people, setting up with the left foot forward. If you are left-handed, my apologies, simply reverse all right and left-handed instructions. Everything is the same, just the other way round.

1. Hitting the bag

It is not unusual for beginners to wonder about the best way to "make a fist" in such a way that they will not hurt the hand, especially the thumb. Most injuries that beginners incur are to the wrist (through failure to keep a straight arm on contact), or to the thumb (through incorrect placement of the thumb).

    Settle hand comfortably into your glove, pulling hard on the wristband to ensure a snug fit. When buying gloves try them on wearing hand-wraps. For this reason (quite apart from the fragrance issue), you need your own bag mitts.

    Close hand, leaving thumb in the "thumbs-up" position.

    Draw thumb tightly down against fingers. Thumb MUST be retained in this position. Failure to do so will almost certainly lead, sooner or later, to injury.

    If this proves problematic, try tailor-made "cut-thumb" style bag mitts, which are generally about the same cost as the orthodox type. A radical alternative would be to cut off the thumb section of your old gloves to see if this provides a solution. As with footwear, never persist with any kit that is uncomfortable. The problem usually just gets worse.

2. The stance

Imagine you are standing on a clock face, your left foot on 12 o'clock and your right foot at twenty past twelve. Try to stay close to this stance, never cross your feet.

Your bodyweight leans minimally forward from the waist. You are not bolt upright but slightly crouched. Your chin is low enough to have a tennis ball trapped underneath it, but your eyes should be on the target. Both elbows are tucked comfortably against the ribs and the right hand is close to the chin. The left hand is held at the same height as the right, but about a foot ahead of it. Arms and legs should feel relaxed: loose limbs travel faster and smoother, so avoid tension at all costs.

3. Movement

All you need to remember when you first start is:

The front foot takes you forwards; the back foot takes you backwards

If you want to go right push off with the left foot

If you want to go left push off with the right foot

Stay on the balls of your feet and practice maintaining good balance as you move around. Do not bounce; move in a sliding fashion, gliding like a ballroom dancer – a tough ballroom dancer.

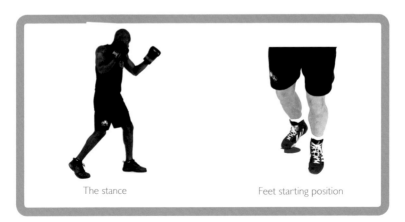

The stance   Feet starting position

The Punches

For the purposes of this exercise we will be using 3 punches: the jab, the straight right (or right cross) and the hook.

The left Jab

This is quite a natural action, delivered sharply and cleanly, more like a spear than a club. Just snap the left glove to the target in a straight line, landing with the knuckle part of the glove. Turn the left hip and shoulder as you do for a little added power. The most important part of throwing a punch is the transfer of weight. When you jab you should use the ball of the right (rear) foot to propel your weight forward, stepping a few inches forward with the left (front) foot; try to picture somebody standing on your right toe as you get the 'feel'. Don't let the back foot come off the ground, you are not going for an 'Eros' look as you finish.

Directly after making contact retract the glove to the basic stance position, keeping the right hand alongside your chin and not allowing it to drop – it now has a job to do…

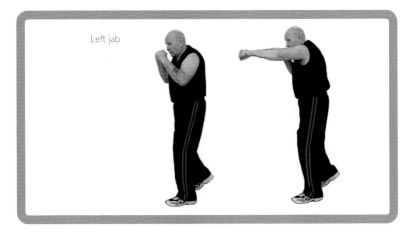

Left jab

The straight right/right cross

This is where you can turn the power on, which is why the 'big' hand stays back instead of leading. This is hitting off your naturally stronger wing and the full satisfying feeling that accompanies it as you zing it into the bag. This is not a spear; this is a trip-hammer. As with the jab you will need the transference of weight, driving off the ball of the right foot, turning the hip and shoulder in the direction of the target. The upper row of knuckles are the hardest part of the hand, so attempt to punch slightly downwards on impact to ensure this part of the hand makes contact first. Stay upright, keeping the shoulders over the hips, to avoid 'reaching' for the target in such a way that the upper body leans forward, which will result in a large loss of power.

When you go forward, take your hips with you. Try not to list over to your left, which is a common error. The left side of your body should allow the right side to pivot, as it acts like a hinge. Do not drop the left hand as you throw the right; keep it alongside your face. Keep chin down and eyes on the target and retract the right glove in the same line as it went out in directly after contact.

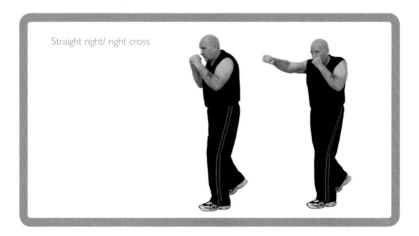

Straight right/ right cross

The hook

The left hand comes back into the action now, with a classic, short, hard punch. To launch the hook, shift your weight to the side you intend to strike from, the left in this case, turning the hip and shoulder slightly away from the target. Your arm is bent at the elbow, at about 90 degrees. The other hand is kept close to the head. By rapidly raising the heel and pivoting the hip of the hitting side simultaneously, make a powerful turn and slam the hand against the target with the upper knuckles leading and the thumb (tucked in tightly) on top at contact. The instant after hitting whip the hand back to the start position, so you could repeat the punch if you wanted to. If you have trouble turning your hips bring the rear foot forward a few inches.

For a right hook simply peel away to your right and then take the same action as you did with the left.

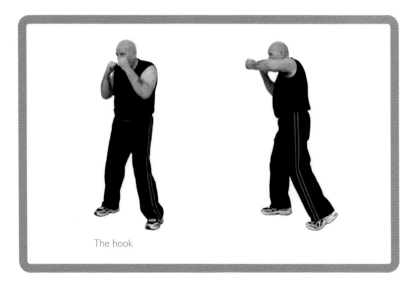

The hook

Shadow Boxing

This is good exercise on its own; it gives you the chance to get used to the footwork and throw all the punches. Only hit when you stop moving; leave hitting on the move to legends like Ali. Don't put too much effort or power into your punches, stay totally relaxed throughout. Don't extend the arms fully or lock your elbows out. Try to keep your foot stance in the '20-past-12' position as you cruise around.

The Activities

For this exercise it is a good idea to stretch the hand and forearm muscles. This is done to protect the elbow and wrist joints and the associated ligaments against the shock of hitting the bag. Run through these stretches after your workout as well.

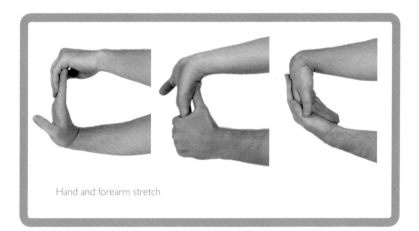

Hand and forearm stretch

	Start with a 5 minute warm-up: skipping, shadow boxing or a combination of both.
	Short stretch (see stretch section) and mobilise joints.
1.	Skipping (will restore your body heat that may have cooled a little during your stretch. See section on skipping if you are new to skipping).
2.	Shadow box (throw jabs, straight rights and hooks from both hands as you move around in the 20 past 12 footwork stance. Only throw punches when you are static, not on the move. Use half power only, boxers use this as a rehearsal and so should you, so do not lock your elbows on the straight punches).
3.	Punch bag (on your first session hit light and fast).
4.	Skip (at an easy pace).
5	Crunches or curl-ups (on the floor or using the Fit-ball).
6	Step-ups (alternate left for 10 and then right for 10).
7.	Squats (with or without weights, to be performed slowly).
8.	Fast skip (get a little speed up for one minute).
9.	Punch bag (here's where you 'get stuck in').
10.	'Box' press-ups if you cannot manage the full version.
11.	Easy jogging (or alternated with a little more pace as you run to and fro).
12.	Punch bag (as before, unload powerfully on this session).
13.	Skip at a relaxed pace for 3 minutes if this is going to be your 'cool down' skip prior to your post exercise long stretch. If you are going to do a second run-through then only skip for two minutes.

Sample combinations

1.	Jab, straight right, left hook, right hook.
2.	Jab, jab, straight right, left hook
3.	Left hook high, left hook low (waist high), right hook
4.	Jab low, jab high, straight right, left hook
5.	Jab, low straight right, left hook, straight right
6.	Jab, left hook, right hook, right hook low.
7.	Jab, jab, right hook, left hook, straight right.

Preparation

You don't want to over-run your allotted time so a large, visible clock would be handy, as most people prefer to remove their watch when wearing bag mitts. This is where a timer with a countdown facility comes in handy, or an egg timer that 'dings' at zero, a stopwatch with an audible alarm, or a watch with an audible alarm. Usually mobile phones have a countdown timer. The one on my Nokia is suitably loud and audible. You need to have one eye on the clock or a device that has an alarm perceptible above the sound of a skipping rope, a bag being walloped or a thumping stereo system.

Have some water standing by, in order to sip as you go and a towel if you think you will need it. I'll be surprised if this little lot doesn't make you sweat.

Am I Too Old?

How old is too old? I hear people of forty tell me they are too old for this kind of training, until they try it, prove themselves wrong and often turn out to be more committed than their younger counterparts. Not too many years ago fitness classes for the over-50s consisted of gentle exercises, much of it performed while seated; a far cry from the friends I know who continue doing martial arts, swim for miles (daily), run 2-3 times every week, cycle prodigious distances and weight train regularly. All of them maintain flexibility by regular stretching.

If you are reasonably fit, disease-free, with no debilitating injuries, full medical clearance and are prepared to take a patient, sensible view about fitness aspirations, there is a great deal of boxing fitness you can participate in and derive benefit from.

A once-a-week session of light skipping, punching bags and pads, and especially weight training and steady jogging should not over-extend elderly people. Consider the vast numbers of 60 and 70 year olds who canter breezily through the London Marathon (and even more in the major American marathons). Flexibility is a must for the older trainer; the maxim "use it or lose it" is apt in this respect.

Moderation is the key. Work comfortably within your limits initially. It is an unfortunate fact that strains and pulls come easily to the more mature person and take what seems an aeon to clear up. Never write yourself off; after all, this form of training should give you renewed confidence and self-esteem. Don't feel self-conscious or worry about what other people think; you will probably gain the grudging admiration of younger trainers around you, who are hoping they will be as fit as you when they get to your age! Take the long view and be content to build up slowly in small but steady increments; you are unlikely to be bored.

> *"Growing old is not for cissies"*
>
> Bette Davis

26. Weight Training for the Over-50s

Weight training is an invaluable training tool for both young and old in that it:

1. Builds strength

2. Improves muscular fitness

3. Burns off excess fat (more than most people realise)

4. Retards osteoporosis by improving bone density

5. Increases metabolic rate, which makes you burn more calories

"Most athletes use strength training as a means of preparing for their sporting life. The same might be said for elderly people, who could include strength training as a means of protecting their quality of life. A number of studies have indicated that the aged exhibit marked increases in muscle strength (40-300%) after 8-12 weeks of training."

('Exercise and Physical Activity in Older People' Meg Morris & Adrian Schoo, BH books).

Safety First

If you are going to start weight training at the gym on either machines or free weights you must have a programme designed for you by a professional instructor, not "a mate who's been doing weights for years." This is not a corner you can cut.

If you elect to train at home with weights, keep it as light as possible, especially if you are a novice. Try to train with a partner in order to assist one another by *spotting* (tracking the movement of weights, or assisting at the beginning and end of the lift to ensure safety).

If weights need to be tightened with an Allen key, spring collar or screw-type collar – check for tightness every time you use them.

Only perform recognised exercises as demonstrated by an instructor or listed in respected manuals, do not feel tempted to improvise or invent moves of your own.

Work slowly – this way you will recruit the maximum amount of muscle fibre. Imagine you are performing the lifts as if underwater. There are no weight training moves that you need to do quickly.

Always keep your back straight. The two most common reasons, in my experience, for people packing-in weight training are a) boredom (they have never upgraded their programme) and b) they hurt their back through bad technique.

Don't be a hero. This is mainly a male thing; the guy who went before you just lifted 50kg, you don't want to look like a wimp by stripping the weight down to your prescribed 20kg. Don't do this – you may do yourself irreparable harm as you will lack the strength or technique to deal with the load. Remember that we all have different needs, lifting light weights is recommended for many aspects of boxing and martial arts training, so don't feel you have to be macho about lifting – do your own thing.

Be patient. We all progress at different rates. Some people show improvement rapidly, others take months and months. Never despair, it always works – just give it time.

27. Free Weights or Machines?

My advice would always be to start with machine weights and then graduate to free weights, with proper instruction from a qualified instructor. Once you have mastered both applications you can devise a workout using elements of each, if you so choose, or change your workout frequently. This is highly advisable, not only to escape boredom, but also to progress with your weight training and fitness rather than hitting a plateau.

Some exercises you may find *difficult* to perform but *never* do an exercise that hurts – it cannot possibly be doing you any good. A decent instructor will find you an alternative. For example, some people have difficulty raising their arms above their heads to perform a shoulder press, usually because of back, shoulder or neck problems. An alternative would be to perform a lateral raise exercise, which will competently exercise the shoulder muscles.

If you are buying weights for the home and are considering a multigym, they are quite a good option, particularly regarding safety, just so long as they are solidly constructed.

On the whole you get what you pay for when buying exercise equipment but multigyms have remained competitively priced for some time now. If you want a high end machine with precision engineering you can pay several thousand pounds; Nautilus (a premier brand) produce a model retailing around the two thousand mark. Closer to most people's pocket is the York Compact, selling for about £199; not bad for a multigym promising to deliver 36 exercise routines, 12 weight levels and up to 60 kilograms of resistance. York also produce multi-gyms and have a reasonable reputation for quality in the industry. Needless to say my 'benchmark' supplier, Argos, have machines priced from £169.99 from Reebok (another redoubtable brand) to £799 from Sportline. As you go up in price the machines become more sophisticated and varied in their scope, but the Compact would suit a first-time buyer who is not too experienced. Size and storage play a huge part as well. A multigym may take up about anything from 20 square feet in space and stand, on average, 6-7 feet high; which, given the fact you have to move around it in safety and comfort means it is on the greedy side for home space. The overall weight of the multigym must also be taken into consideration. I would recommend a concrete floor for place of installation, unless you have incredibly strong floorboards and the people who dwell below you are either understanding and easygoing, or hard of hearing.

Free weights can also take up a lot of space, especially if you add a bench and a barbell support, or a combination of both, and a rack to keep your weights tidy, to prevent your loved ones tumbling over them in the dark.

If you intend to train indoors you may be better off with plastic-coated dumbbells or plates; hard-core metal equipment is more suited to the shed or garage, especially if there are floorboards. There still exist shops that sell purely weight training equipment, some under a franchise such as Weider, where the equipment choice is wide and the opportunity to talk to somebody with specific experience to help you with your purchases can be invaluable. Weigh up the cost of buying from a specialist store alongside buying from Argos, Ebay or other web sites where no informative assistance is forthcoming. I have usually found the customer service in these stores to be first-rate; unfortunately, as one owner informed me, many only exist on the strength of their supplement sales.

If you are just starting up, then a free weight set, consisting of a barbell and associated plates and a pair of dumbbells (costing about £30 from York, Weider and others) will get you on the road to muscular improvement. You do not need anything heavier than a total of 35 kilograms from the sum total of the complete kit. Your initial workout will be lugging it home from the store.

A bench will come in handy to give more variety to your workout and is essential for chest press and pectoral flyes. I picked my bench up from a second-hand exercise equipment seller (where a wide variety of discarded kit was piled up in a barn). It cost £15 and with a clean-up and a coat of Hammerite paint on the iron frame it is as good as new, in which case it would cost three times that price. These outlets are usually to be located in the Yellow Pages. They tend not to go in for websites but they are a haven for browsing for home equipment as they buy from gyms who are upgrading their facilities and you can even haggle with them.

The Choice at the Gym

A qualified instructor who is starting you on a weights programme will in all probability show you how to operate the machine weights initially, as they are easier and safer. Once you are competent and confident you should ask him or her to show you how to use free weights safely and with correct technique. Let the instructor know why you are doing weight training and your aims, to allow him or her to tailor the workout to your personal needs. Once you are assured on both, there is a wealth of written material to help you with your progress and to help with diversity. Most people in my experience throw their hand in for one of two reasons:

1. Boredom – usually because they never change their workout

2. Pain – hurting their back or similar (in most cases through bad technique, or over-lifting beyond their capability).

Don't fall prey to either of the above by:

1. Changing your workout regularly.

2. If you are unsure about what weight to lift – always aim low, err on the side of caution.

For and against machine weights

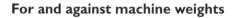

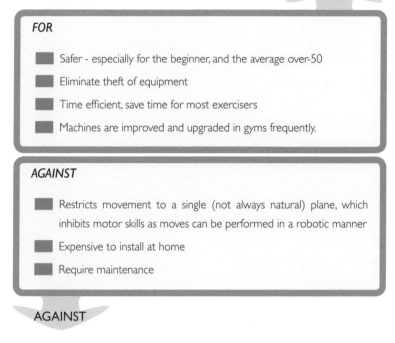

FOR

■ Safer - especially for the beginner, and the average over-50

■ Eliminate theft of equipment

■ Time efficient, save time for most exercisers

■ Machines are improved and upgraded in gyms frequently.

AGAINST

■ Restricts movement to a single (not always natural) plane, which inhibits motor skills as moves can be performed in a robotic manner

■ Expensive to install at home

■ Require maintenance

AGAINST

For and against freeweights

FOR

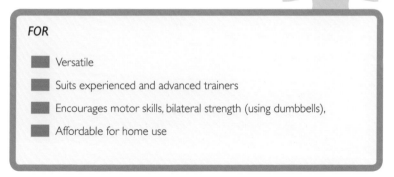

FOR

■ Versatile

■ Suits experienced and advanced trainers

■ Encourages motor skills, bilateral strength (using dumbbells),

■ Affordable for home use

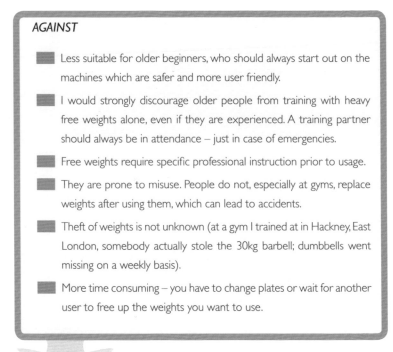

AGAINST

■ Less suitable for older beginners, who should always start out on the machines which are safer and more user friendly.

■ I would strongly discourage older people from training with heavy free weights alone, even if they are experienced. A training partner should always be in attendance – just in case of emergencies.

■ Free weights require specific professional instruction prior to usage.

■ They are prone to misuse. People do not, especially at gyms, replace weights after using them, which can lead to accidents.

■ Theft of weights is not unknown (at a gym I trained at in Hackney, East London, somebody actually stole the 30kg barbell; dumbbells went missing on a weekly basis).

■ More time consuming – you have to change plates or wait for another user to free up the weights you want to use.

AGAINST

In summing up I would stress that the older trainer, especially the novice, is always better off starting with (and probably staying with) machine weights. These machines improve all the time and are very user-friendly.

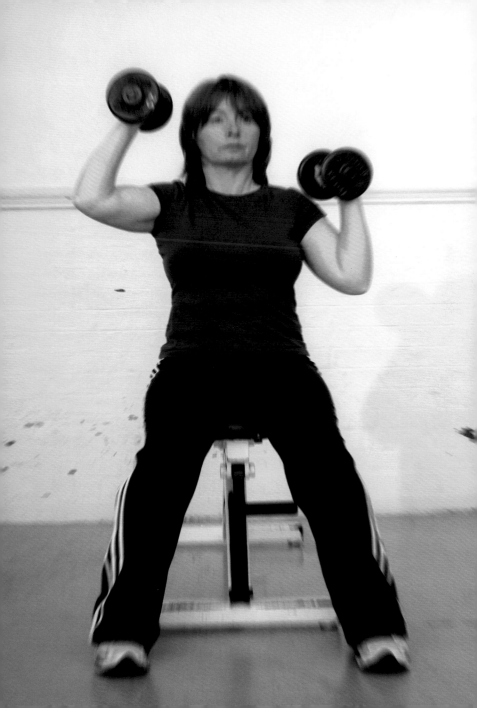

28. Weights Machine Workout

The following workout is for the whole body and can be done up to three times a week, but never on consecutive days as your body needs the following day after the workout for rest, recovery and adaptation. If you adhere to the programme you will almost certainly progress, but this is dependent on your 'staying on the wagon'. The F.I.T principle (frequency, intensity, time spent) applies here. Your improvements hinge on how often and how hard you work.

If you are a newcomer to the gym a qualified instructor should show you how to operate the machines safely and slowly. The exercises are set in order for opposite muscles to work one after the other. The muscles involved are referred to as:

The Agonist

Also called 'The Prime Mover' (the main muscle being exercised)

The Antagonist

The muscle on the opposite side of a joint, which must relax to allow the prime mover to contract. An example is where the bicep 'curls' towards the shoulder and the tricep, at the back of the upper arm, relaxes.

Weight training as performed in this workout is a form of *isotonic training*. In other words, muscles have a concentric action, such as a 'bicep curl' (where the muscle shortens) and an eccentric action, when the arm uncurls back to the original position (lengthens). The eccentric phase, the lowering or unfurling action, is of more importance than the concentric, as more strength gain is acquired by slow, steady eccentric training.

The slower you work the more muscle fibre you can recruit for the task.

The workout I have selected is built around the "10 Rep Max" system, a tried and tested formula that usually suits beginners, but which many people continue with for years, their only changes being to the weight they work with.

Basically the first repetition should be fairly easy but the ninth and tenth a little challenging. Dismiss any ideas that if it doesn't hurt it isn't doing any good. If it does hurt – STOP! You are overdoing it, or doing it wrong.

Use the workout below once you have discovered what weights relate to the principle of the 10 Rep Max. Always err on the side of safety; aim low and let caution be your watchword if you want to get out of bed the following day.

Always leave your arms to the last. If you work them hard in an isolated form they will not give the desired support as secondary movers with regard to the chest and back exercises. I have included abdominals only once, but as you get fitter you can intersperse your abs work between other exercises.

Do not move on to the next exercise until you have completed 2-3 sets. This is not circuit training (you progress in the following fashion):

Example:

Bench press set 1, rest 30-60 seconds; bench press set 2, rest 30-60 seconds; bench press set 3, rest 30-60 seconds. Now move on to lat pull downs in the same pattern.

- Level 1: Start with one set of 10 repetitions for the first 5 workouts.

- Level 2: Start with 2 sets of 10 reps; after 10 workouts move on to 3 sets of 10 reps.

- Levels 3 and 4: Start with 3 sets of 10 reps; increase weights rather than doing more than 3 sets of 10 reps.

Weights machine workout

(Fill in the weights column as you train)

Aerobic warm up for 5 minutes: cycle, row, jog, skip etc..						
Short stretch and mobilisation						
Rest for 30-60 secs between sets, according to how strenuous you found the last set.						
Order	Body part	Exercise	Machine	Sets	Reps	Weight
1.	Pectorals	Pectoral flyes	Pectoral deck machine	2-3	10	
2.	Chest	Bench press	Chest press machine	2-3	10	
3.	Back	Lat pull downs	Lat pull-down machine	2-3	10	
4.	Shoulders	Shoulder press	Shoulder press machine	2-3	10	
5.	Abdominals	Crunches	Seated crunch machine	2-3	10	
6.	Quadriceps	Leg extensions	Leg extension machine	2-3	10	
7.	Hamstrings	Leg curls	Seated/lying leg curl machine	2-3	10	
8.	Calf	Seated/standing calf raise	Calf raise machine	2-3	10	
(Omit if you have any history of calf or Achilles injuries or strains)						
9.	Biceps	Bicep curls	Curl machine or low pulley station	2-3	10	
10.	Triceps	Tricep pushdowns	High pulley station	2-3	10	
Warm down with 5 minutes of aerobic exercise, followed by a long stretch						

The shorter weights machine workout

You were stuck in traffic, delayed at the office or got a puncture and now you don't have time to do a full workout – or do you? If this is the case go with the abridged (but still beneficial) version. At least you will work the large, essential muscle groups – the chest, back and legs. All sense of guilt and self-disgust is thereby removed.

Warm-up, stretch and mobilise as before						
Order	Body part	Exercise	Exercise machine	Sets	Reps	Weight
1.	Chest	Bench press	Chest press machine	2-3	10	
2.	Back	Lat pull downs	Lat pull-down machine	2-3	10	
3.	Quadriceps	Leg extensions	Leg extension machine	2-3	10	
4.	Hamstrings	Leg curls	Seated/ lying leg curl machine	2-3	10	
Then warm down and do long stretch as above						

Substitute exercise machines

As not all gyms have the same equipment, the following are alternative exercises, which in most cases are equally as effective.

Body part	Exercise machine	Substitute
Chest	Seated chest press machine	Bench press
Back	Seated row machine	Lat pull down machine
Back	High pulley	Lat pull downs
Chest and legs	Smith Machine	a) flat for bench press b) inclined for upper chest c) declined for lower chest d) can also be used for squats if no leg stations available
Quads	Leg press machine	Leg extension machine
Upper back and rear of shoulders (trapezius and posterior deltoids)	Low pulley upright rows – well worth adding to the above workout.	Shoulder press machine
Biceps (in isolation)	'Preacher' station	Curl machine
Shoulders – middle and front of shoulders (medial and anterior deltoids)	Low pulley lateral raises	Shoulder press machine

All of the above are worth becoming familiar with; if you use the same machines all the time it can grow tedious. Switching to new apparatus helps bring some variety and helps to challenge your muscles. Just as your muscles get comfortable doing it one way, shake them out of their lethargy and make them learn a new skill.

Never use apparatus on which you have not received instruction. Simply ask one of the instructors how to use the machine. Even if they are busy they will generally schedule a time for you to come in to try the machine in safety.

Steer Clear!

If you are over 50 I would personally advise *against* using the following machines:

Neck machines:

I haven't seen one of these rascals for a while, but there is an attachment, referred to as the *head harness* to put around your head in order to 'strengthen' your neck.

Charles Lynch, who pioneered lynching, and the inventor of this device must have gone to school together.

Machine Trunk Rotations

In this exercise the user, who I feel I should refer to as 'the victim', stands on a circular *swivel plate* and holds on to the t-shaped handle. The intention is to work the obliques by rotating on the swivelling plate. It can be performed reasonably safely by an experienced trainer, but full rotation of the spine is fraught with all sorts of danger with regard to back injury – give this one a miss.

Leg Press 'Variations'

Some well-meaning person may inform you that if you place your toes on the edge of the plate of a leg press machine you can rock it to and fro to work your calf muscles. I do not recommend this – one false slip, or a moment of inattention and you could finish up a similar height to Toulouse-Lautrec. Keep your feet a shoulder-width apart in the middle of the plate – this is a heavy machine.

Do look out for

Keiser Machinery (Keiser Pneumatic Technology)

This equipment is quite unique and the most user-friendly apparatus. It doesn't require the user to shift metal plates, pulleys or chains, but instead resistance is provided by a central compressor. The user adjusts the station to exactly the weight he wants to work with, increasing the pressure by pressing down on the right hand button, or decreasing it by pressing down on the left hand button. Pressing both buttons simultaneously will reset the repetition counter, so don't worry if you loose count – the machine keeps score!

The reason it is appealing to the older user is that most weights machines need an initial drive to get the stack started, but the compressor system makes sure the effort is consistent throughout the concentric and eccentric phases.

The Keiser people have put a lot of research into training for mature folk, as they realised that more and more older people want to train but need user-friendly facilities. I would still combine a free weights workout on another day, but if you used only this machinery I am sure most people would make strength gains of some degree.

Where there is Keiser equipment, there is usually a layout referred to as the 'Keiser X-Press Training Circuit': weights stations are interspersed with cardio stations (usually static cycles or rowers) and there is opportunity to stretch between stations. Cardio work, weight training and stretching are performed in rotation.

The main drawback with this excellent equipment is its lack of availability; most gyms in Britain still haven't caught onto the 'grey pound'. It would appear that the fitness industry still has its sights firmly set on the under 40's. The other small niggle is that the weights are in pounds, not kilos, so if you are used to kilos you might need to pop a conversion chart in your bag.

If you do have access to Keiser equipment, use the machines in this order:

    Chest press

    Lat pull downs

- Shoulder press

- Leg extension

- Leg curl

- Tricep press downs

- Bicep curl station

- Seated Abdominal crunch station - can be used between sets of other stations.

- Warm-up, stretches and cool down, as per regular weights workout.

29. The Home Multigym Workout

Remember work slowly!

Always work slowly; the more slowly you work the better your technique will be, and the more muscle fibre you will involve. Working slowly is extremely important if you are a newcomer to your machinery (having just taken it out of the box, taken a day to assemble it and are chomping at the bit to get cracking). If for no better reason than your personal safety, always work slowly and under control; it is the most assured way of achieving a positive result.

Always try to exhale on the major exertion.

When lifting a bar, slowly count to three, pause at the top of the lift for three seconds and then count to three slowly as you lower the bar.

Always ensure you are comfortable before starting the first rep, if you are not comfortable at this stage, be assured it's only going to become worse as you progress. Take time to settle into position first for confident training.

It is absolutely essential to restrain the lowering (eccentric) phase of the exercise – this has more effect on your training than the lifting (concentric) phase, strange as this may seem.

How Much Weight?

If you do not know how much weight you can lift in each of the following exercises, take my advice and aim low! Starting out with a low weight (the lowest possible if you are a beginner) will achieve the following:

1. You will be a lot less likely to cause injury.

2. You will understand, appreciate and control what you are trying to achieve.

3. You will gradually build up your confidence in your ability to make strength gains.

Order of Exercises

Flyes on "pec deck" (chest muscles)

Bring the padded plates together; get used to synchronising them to arrive in the centre at the same speed and time! Resist the urge to clash them together like cymbals; halt their progress when they are about an inch apart. In doing so, you will be unlikely to introduce a rebounding effect but will improve your motor skills.

Bench press (chest muscles)

Make sure your head is on the bench and not overhanging the end in any way. Your hands, gripping the handles, should be either side of your chest. If your back doesn't feel flat against the bench, or is not totally comfortable, bend your knees and put your feet up on the bench. Extend your arms fully, keeping your wrists flat and straight; don't bend your wrists as this will place excessive stress on them.

Lat (latissimus dorsi) pull downs (back muscles)

Sit facing the machine; if there is a restraint pad, tuck your knees under it. Take a wide grip, holding the bar near the ends. Pull the bar down slowly, arching your back and retracting your elbows until the bar is level with your chest. Do not allow the bar to return under its own steam, restrain it to produce a controlled return of the bar until your arms are extended upwards. It is a safety hazard, as well as incorrect procedure, to allow the bar to fly back on its own with minimal restraint.

Upright rows (rear of shoulders and back)

Take the bar from the low pulley setting at the foot of the stack and pull it up until it is in front of your thighs. Ideally your hands should be about one foot apart. Slowly pull the bar straight up to chin height, raising your elbows to shoulder height as you do so. Return the bar smoothly to the start position.

Seated rows (back muscles)

Sit facing the low pulley. If you have a V-bar or Double-D bar attachment use this, if not use the shortest bar available. Ensuring your feet are in a stable position, lean forward so that your head is above your knees, or as far forward as is comfortable. Arch your back as you pull the bar back to reach your mid-section, with the elbows pulled back past your body.

Shoulder press (shoulder muscles)

Grasp handles and raise vertically, ensuring your wrists stay flat and straight; do not bend your wrists as doing so will place excessive stress on them. Keep head up, facing directly ahead. Lower the weight slowly.

Low pulley lateral raise (shoulder muscles)

Grasp the pulley handle with one hand and steady yourself by holding the multigym frame with the other hand, to steady yourself. Start out with head up, feet shoulder-width apart and the handle at thigh level. Extend your arm outwards to shoulder-height in a slow, controlled manner. Restrain the return.

Leg extensions (thigh muscles / quads)

Seated with the front of your ankles against the pads of the leg extension machine, slowly raise your legs to the horizontal (do not kick upwards) and then return under restraint. Do not allow the weight to drop, which is all too easy to do. You don't want to become a 'swinger', whipping the weight up and down.

Seated leg curls (hamstrings)

Do this exercise straight after your leg extensions. Place the back of your ankles on the pads and adjust the restraint bar across your thighs slowly drive them down and back as far as they will go. Return to horizontal position slowly.

Lying leg curls (hamstrings)

Some multi-gyms provide a leg curl station that requires you to perform the exercise lying down. Lie face down but with your head raised and your ankles against the pads. Grasp the bench on each side (or handles if they are provided) and bring your feet upward and curl them towards the body, getting your heels as close to your backside as you can manage.

(Both forms of leg curl are equally effective in achieving results, but the 'lying' form tends to work the calf muscle in addition to the hamstring.)

Tricep press-downs (rear of upper arms – triceps)

Use the same long bar as in 'lat pull downs' with a close grip, hands on top of the bar, 6-8 inches apart. If you have a shorter straight bar, or better still, a 'Triceps V-rope' attachment, a length of thick rope formed in a 'v' with large rubber knobs at the ends to prevent the hands sliding off. These are reasonably cheap and highly beneficial for this exercise.

To help with stability, stand with feet shoulder-width apart and upper body leaning forward slightly. It is very important to keep the upper arm as still as possible as you slowly press the weight down. Starting position should be just below the chest and finish position should level with the thighs as you fully extend your arms. Keep as still as you can, don't rock 'n' roll to complete the movement, if you are doing this you have too much weight for correct technique.

Bicep cable curls (front of upper arms – biceps)

Start with the bar, attached to the low pulley station, across your thighs. Slowly curl the bar towards your chest, using only your lower arms. Do not force the bar upward by rocking your body backward. If you have to pull your head and shoulders back to lift the weight then it is too heavy; only use as much weight as you can curl solely with lower arm movement.

A specific piece of equipment for this exercise is the 'curl bar', which you attach to the low pulley station and allows a greater range of movement.

Leg Press - a word of warning

Avoid using excessive weight on the leg press as it can put strain on the sacroiliac joint, which can cause lower back pain, or even vertibrate displacement. Unless you are an experienced weight trainer, keep to a moderate weight load on this excellent piece of equipment, which, used correctly, is terrific for strengthening the upper leg muscles and glutes. You must keep your backside firmly in the seat, your back against the pad and your feet squarely in the middle of the plate, roughly shoulder-width apart. Start with knees bent at a right angle and push the plate away slowly and smoothly and restrain the return, as opposed to letting it swing back on its own.

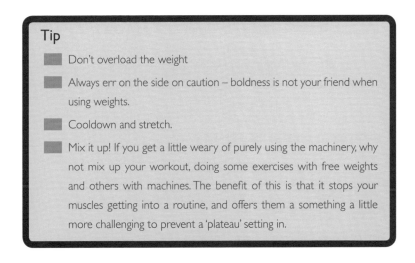

Tip

- Don't overload the weight

- Always err on the side on caution – boldness is not your friend when using weights.

- Cooldown and stretch.

- Mix it up! If you get a little weary of purely using the machinery, why not mix up your workout, doing some exercises with free weights and others with machines. The benefit of this is that it stops your muscles getting into a routine, and offers them a something a little more challenging to prevent a 'plateau' setting in.

30. Weight Training: Free Weights

The Gym or Home Workout

Kit required:

Free weights, bench, chair (unless bench folds into seated position).

Warm up, stretches and mobilisation

5 minutes skipping, cycling, rowing or similar to raise your temperature and warm your muscles, as this will prepare you for the exercise ahead and reduce the risk of injury (see warm-up and warm down sections).

> ### Tip
> Don't use step machines for warm-ups as it can place great emphasis on your (cold) calf muscles resulting in soreness. Choose something that warms up the large muscle groups.

The 'one minute' stretch (ok, just over one minute)

A 5 minute warm-up will only be adequate to allow you a short standing stretch – any excessive stretching at this stage could be harmful and retrogressive. All these stretches should be held for 6-8 seconds.

Perform stretches for:

Shoulders, back, chest, hamstrings, quads, calf muscles (see pages 52-55)

Mobilisation

So on to the mobilisation stage, where we attempt to get some synovial fluid (the juice that oils our joints) into the joints. Youngsters don't need too much of this, but it's important for seniors, and doesn't take more than about a minute.

Neck: Look over your shoulder, drop your chin to gaze at the ground as you slowly turn to look over the other shoulder. Repeat twice.

Shoulders: Slowly rotate your arms three times forward and three back.

Knees: Support your upper body and raise your leg behind you until parallel with the ground a few times. Repeat with other leg.

Ankles: Slowly rotate each ankle in circles three or four times in each direction.

Wrists: Support your arm as you rotate each wrist a few times in each direction. Conclude by shaking fingers as if flicking water from them.

Now you are ready!

Remember your breathing pattern:

Never hold your breath.

Inhale on the easier downward phase.

Exhale on the harder lifting phases; remember my crude, but effective maxim: *Blow on the effort.*

Workout 1: Weights

Equipment required:

Free weights, bench, chair (unless using folding bench, which allows upright supported seated position) and floor mat.

Apparatus for warm-up: exercise cycle or skipping rope. Simply running on the spot or shadow-boxing tends to lose its appeal after several sessions.

Additional: water (sip as you train), towel.

The exercises

The exercises are arranged in such a way that the biceps and triceps are not emphasised consecutively, the reason being that smaller muscles need to recover in order to assist the larger muscle exercises. For this reason the arms are trained last, being the smallest muscle group to be exercised.

All levels should rest for 30 seconds between each set but this can be lengthened for Level 1 trainers for up to 60 seconds.

Remember this workout must not be carried out on consecutive days, as your muscles need time to adapt to the overload incurred during the session and they can only do this at rest. Working on consecutive days will cause muscular pain bad enough to deter you from wanting to ever train again – take the word of a fool who once tried it in his ignorance. Nobody I know has made this mistake twice. Less is more in progressive weight development.

Suggested frequency:

Level 1: twice a week, preferably with a two day gap.

Level 2: 2-3 times in an 8 day period.*

Levels 3 & 4: ideally 3 times in an 8 day period.*

* I have made it an '8 day week' to make it easier to take the weekend off as your rest time, which I know will suit some people. It also, hopefully, relieves the pressure of trying to squeeze 3 sessions into a week, and the sense of failure when you can't fit it in.

When to do 'the Abs'

Levels 1 & 2:

At conclusion of weights exercises.

Levels 3 & 4:

Inserted between weights exercises, for example after concluding each exercise perform 1 set of abs.

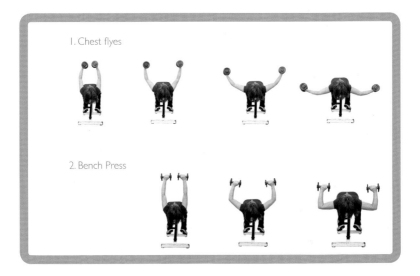

1. Chest flyes

2. Bench Press

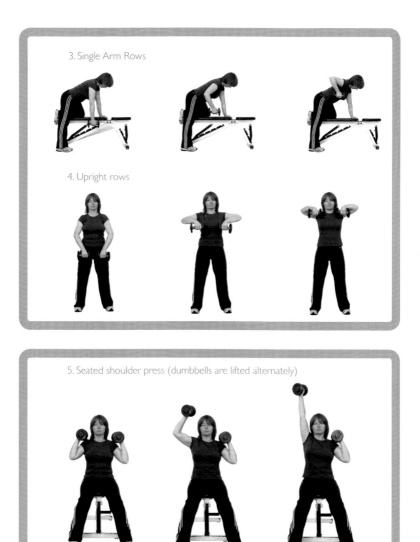

3. Single Arm Rows

4. Upright rows

5. Seated shoulder press (dumbbells are lifted alternately)

6. Lateral Raise

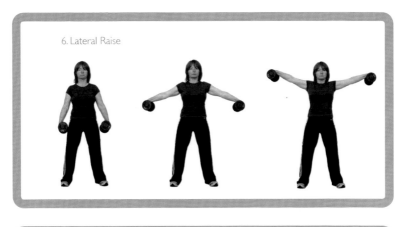

7. Squats with weights

8. Lunges with weights

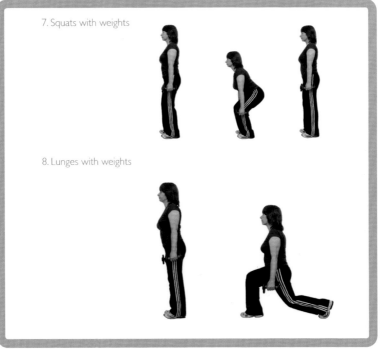

9. Step-ups with weights

10. Deadlifts

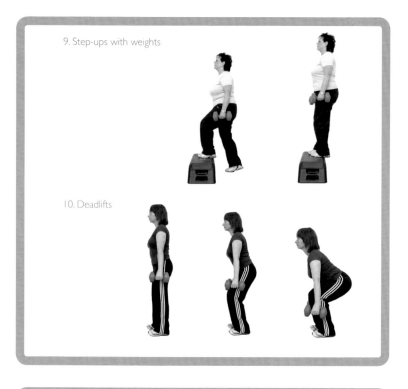

11. Seated dumbbell curls

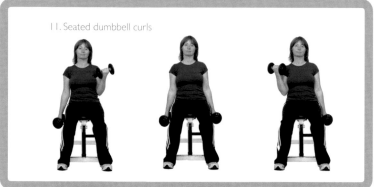

234

12. Bench dips

13. Tricep kickbacks

14. Seated dumbbell extensions

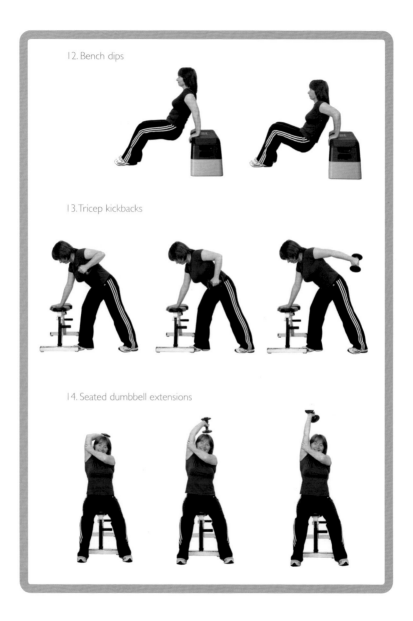

15. Curl ups

16. Standing Twists

17. Reverse curls

18. Crunches with feet raised

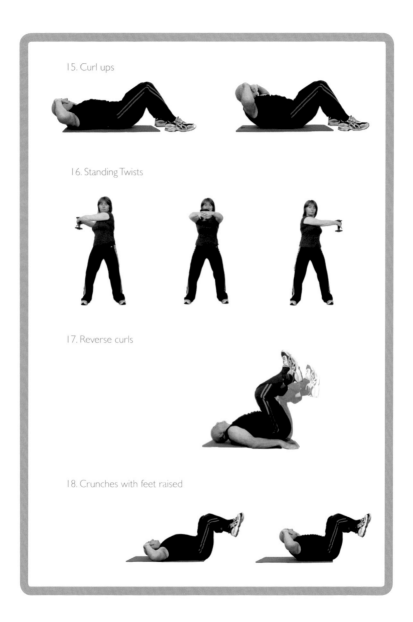

19. Russian twists

20. "The Plank"

21. "The Side Plank"

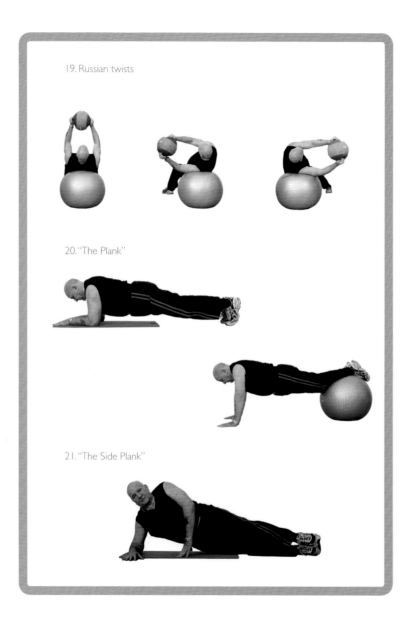

Order	Level	Exercise	Body part	Sets & repetitions
1.	Levels 2,3 & 4 (level 1 can skip this)	Chest flyes	Chest	2 sets of 10 reps
2.	Level 1	Bench press	Chest	2 sets of 10 reps
	Levels 2,3 & 4			3 sets of 10 reps
3.	Level 1	Single arm rows	Back	2 sets of 10 reps each side
	Levels 2,3 & 4			3 sets of 10 reps each side
4.	Level 1	Upright rows	Upper back & rear of shoulders	2 sets of 10 reps
5.	Level 1	Seated shoulder press (dumbbells are lifted alternately)	Shoulders	2 sets of 10 reps (in total)
	Level 2			3 sets of 16 reps (in total)
	Levels 3 & 4		3 sets of 20 reps (in total)	
6.	Levels 3 & 4 only	Lateral raise	Shoulders	3 sets of 10 reps
7.	Level 1	Squats (with light weights)	Thigh and buttocks	2 sets of 10 reps
	Level 2	Moderate weights	2 sets of 10 reps	
	Level 3	Fairly heavy weight	3 sets of 10 reps	
	Level 4	Tolerably heavy weights	3 sets of 10 reps	
8.	Levels 2,3 & 4 only	Lunges	Buttocks, quads, hamstrings – according to stride length	
	Level 2	No weights – arms out for balance, like tightrope walker		2 sets of 10 reps

(Photocopiable page © Ian Oliver 2006)

	Level 3	Light weights	3 sets of 10 reps	
	Level 4	Fairly heavy weights	3 sets of 10 reps	
	An alternative to squats are step-ups, which put less emphasis on the knee.			
9.	Level 1	Step-ups (without weights)	Quads, hamstrings and glutes – according to height of box	2 sets of 10 step-ups on each leg
	Level 2	Without weights or with light weights		3 x sets of 10 step-ups on each leg
	Level 3	With moderately heavy weights		3 x sets of 10 step-ups on each leg
	Level 4	With tolerably heavy weights		3 x sets of 10 step-ups on each leg

(Photocopiable page © Ian Oliver 2006)

Having completed this session, congratulate yourself on your prowess and then prepare for the final two stages of your session; the warm-down and the warm-down stretch.

The Warm-Down

The warm-down is a vital part of the workout; sudden cessation of exercise can be harmful to the heart. Five minutes of light aerobic exercise will gradually return your heart to a more restful state. It serves to get the blood returning to your heart from the large muscles, particularly the legs, where it can have a tendency to 'pool'. Take it easy as you perform this stage and combine getting your breathing back to normal at the same time as your body temperature cools. It is generally accepted that the warm-down helps with the elimination of metabolic waste. The cooling down phase can be 5-10 minutes according to how hard you feel you worked.

Warm-Down Stretches.

Your muscles are now enriched with a copious supply of blood and oxygen, so they can now have a good stretch, lying down if this is comfortable for you. Flop out on your mat, get your breath back and then proceed with the following stretches:

The last stage of your cool-down is passive but something you need and deserve is a cool (not hot) shower, if not a cool bath.

If, by chance, you have a home sauna, this would *not* be the time to use it – your body is trying to cool down and an opposing force such as a sauna, steam room or hot bath will cause a conflict, which could make you feel unwell.

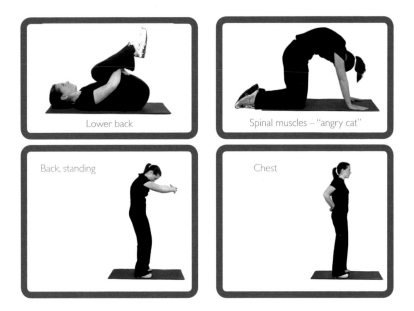

Lower back

Spinal muscles – "angry cat"

Back, standing

Chest

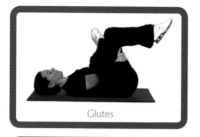

Glutes

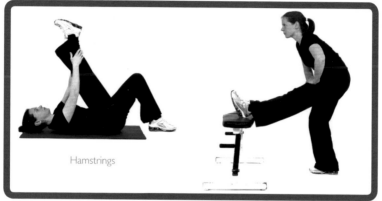

Hamstrings

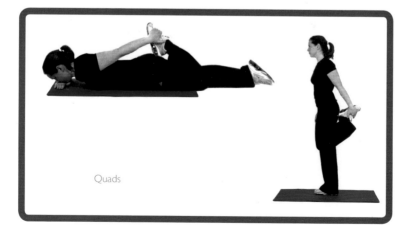

Quads

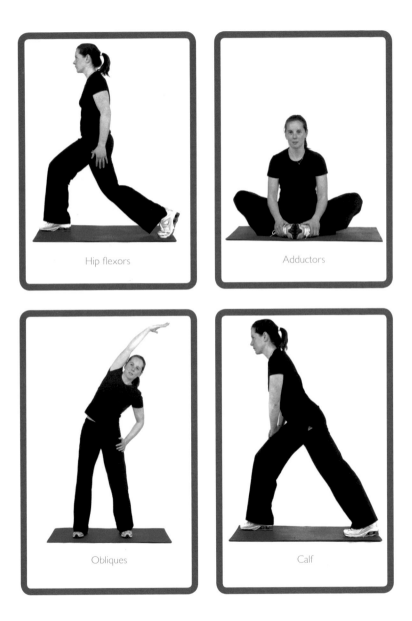

Hip flexors

Adductors

Obliques

Calf

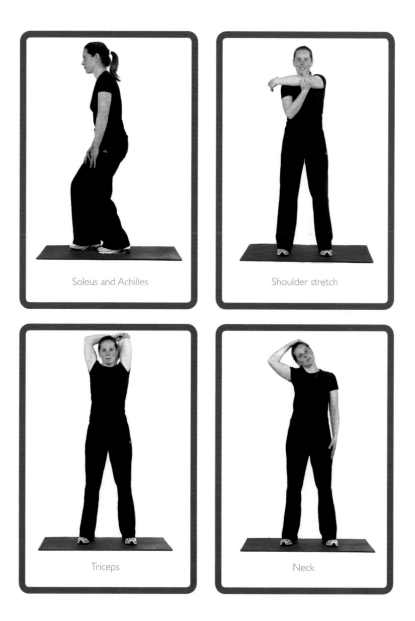

Soleus and Achilles

Shoulder stretch

Triceps

Neck

31. Weights: Split Routine

While the workout prescribed in the previous chapter advises rest on the following day, if you split the body parts over two days (i.e. upper body on one day and then legs on the next) this will not interfere with your rest. It can thus be performed over two, three or four days. Slight variation could allow training to take place on 5-6 days, but I consider everybody needs at least one day off from weights.

This is taking your training to the next level and is quite demanding; I would only advise those training at level 4 to attempt it, but anybody who is training the all-body workout on level 3 could consider moving up to try the following routine. The sample routine shown is a suggested two-way split, suitable for consecutive days.

Suggested Split Routine for 2,3 or 4 days

Level 4 only, or level 3 weight-trainers of over 6 months

Free weights or machines – your choice.

All days

Before: Warm-up, stretch and mobilise joints as before.

After: cool down, long stretch

Day 1 and 3

Flyes

- Bench press

- Lat pull downs (or single arm rows)

- Bicep curls

- Tricep press downs (or tricep dumbbell press)

- Abs work – reverse curls, plank

Day 2 and 4

- Squats

- Lunges

- Or leg extensions and leg curls

- Upright rows

- Shoulder press

- Lateral raise

- Front raise

- Calf raise

- Abs work – crunches, side plank

From routines such as the above you could quite easily divide your muscles into three or four groups, without causing a consecutive day conflict. However, I would advise to start out with a two-way split to gain experience of your individual requirements and training opportunities, before trying to fit more routines in.

32. Women and Weights

The first thing the majority of women tell me when we set out to design a weight training programme is, "I don't want to get big." So, it's all good news – you won't. Look around at the guys in the gym, knocking themselves out lifting and grunting in order to bulk up, look at the trouble they have, having to struggle with huge dumbbells and eat like a horse, and still taking years to develop bigger muscles – and *they* have high levels of testosterone (the male sex hormone). Your low levels of testosterone prevent you from gaining sizeable, masculine-looking muscles, just normal sized firm, sleek-looking muscles.

What weight training will do, additionally, is give you an increase of strength and endurance, and improve your bone density, hopefully reducing the risk of osteoporosis, the causes of which are generally considered to be:

1. Lack of oestrogen or androgens

2. Nutritional deficiency

3. Lack of activity

At the Gym

Never feel inhibited or uncomfortable in the weights area, if the gym has an intimidating atmosphere in the weights section, find a "women-friendly" (i.e. normal) gym; there are enough of them to choose from. Go and view the gym the time you would intend to train to check how crowded it is, and ensure they will provide a qualified instructor to design you a personal programme to show you how to perform the exercises safely and correctly. As an instructor, I was always taught to give clients "their space," and never ever to touch them unless you thought they were going to hurt themselves. We were told never to push or pull people into position; if they were doing an exercise wrong – show them as many times as it takes for them to get it right. Ladies, if your instructor is a little too "handy", over-familiar, or has a tendency to pucker your skin from his garlic-breath – give him his marching papers. If you are paying for a service, then get the service you want and deserve.

33.Studio Classes and the Older Adult

By Victoria Mose, Senior Instructor, YMCA Training and Development Dept.

Gone are the days of Jane Fonda's 'no pain, no gain' ethos. Instructor-led studio classes are now extremely diverse and offer something for everyone. Classes range from group indoor cycling to traditional high/low aerobics and pilates.

The key is finding a selection of classes that work for you. Your instructor should be approachable and make time to talk to you before and after the class, especially if you are a newcomer. If the instructor doesn't bother to provide feedback then find another class or teacher.

Avoid classes that are billed as advanced or *high intensity*. Look for mixed level classes, which offer a variety of exercise options. Don't be put off by 'new' classes, such as Pilates or Body Balance; these classes can offer excellent toning and flexibility benefits. Variety is essential, so avoid going to the same class all the time. Your health and fitness gains will more effective if you attempt new classes occasionally.

Don't be afraid – the studio may have been taken over by thongs and leg-warmers, but there really is a place for everyone.

Whatever your fitness experience level, a good gym will have a range of classes to suit most people, regardless of age.

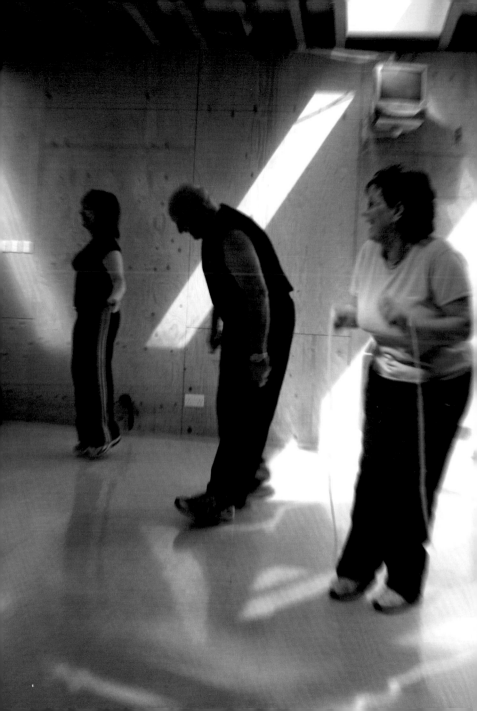

34. Pilates

The man who gave the Pilates Method its name, Joseph Hubertus Pilates, was quite a character. Interned on the Isle of Man during World War I as a German national living in England, he worked as a hospital orderly, treating injured patients and developing rehabilitation techniques which would later form the base of his method. When he moved to New York city in the 1920s, he set up his first studio, offering body conditioning, which became increasingly popular with dancers, as it still remains to this day. He was patronized by dance luminaries and his method was picked up by Hollywood, where it remains popular today. Like every exercise system that succeeds in America, it has reached our shores, albeit considerably later.

It has been popular in Britain for many years now, appealing to people who want a more cerebral exercise than the 'aerobics' variety, and one that does not require jumpy or vigorous movements. Pilates is considered to have a mind and body approach, which will always have an appeal to a large section of the public.

Core aims behind Pilates:

Create/increase balance between strength and flexibility

Improve muscular strength and tone

Improve stability

Improve co-ordination

Improve posture and stance

Improve suppleness

Relieves stress

Pilates uses the core postural muscles to provide strong support for the spine. Emphasis is placed on alignment and posture to alleviate and counteract back problems. This is achieved by:

- Mental focus to improve muscle control and movement efficiency and proficiency

- Being made aware of neutral spine alignment, being made aware of correct stance and posture

- Developing the deep muscles of the abdomen and back

- Developing improved breathing technique and mental focus

- Developing length, strength and flexibility in muscles

Pilates' popularity has been in classes where participants need nothing more than a floor mat, but equipment in Pilates studios is far more complex and you would not usually find this kind of equipment in ordinary gyms. Studios with this apparatus normally specialise in building specific programmes on a one-to-one basis. A session can last between 60-90 minutes, and could cost between £15 to £150 per session.

Mat exercises

This is the most accessible and common form of Pilates. Most of the larger health clubs have caught on to the popularity of alternative exercise and met the demand in a form that will have common appeal. Classes go through a series of exercises to develop strength and flexibility, slowly and under control.

This is not a 'sweaty' class, and seniors attending their initial class are advised, particularly if the studio has air conditioning, to wear something warm, but not bulky.

Authentic and 'modern' pilates

The aficionados of the founder's ethos and methodology would not fully approve, I am sure, of the 'new' form of Pilates, which has brought it to the masses, but no more so than a pro boxing gym would approve of 'Boxercise'. It is nevertheless undeniable that the latest forms, using balls, hoops and mats, has given it wide appeal and saved a lot of back pain. I cannot believe that Joseph Pilates, the ex-circus performer, ex-boxer, self-defence instructor, wartime intern and hospital orderly would have disapproved.

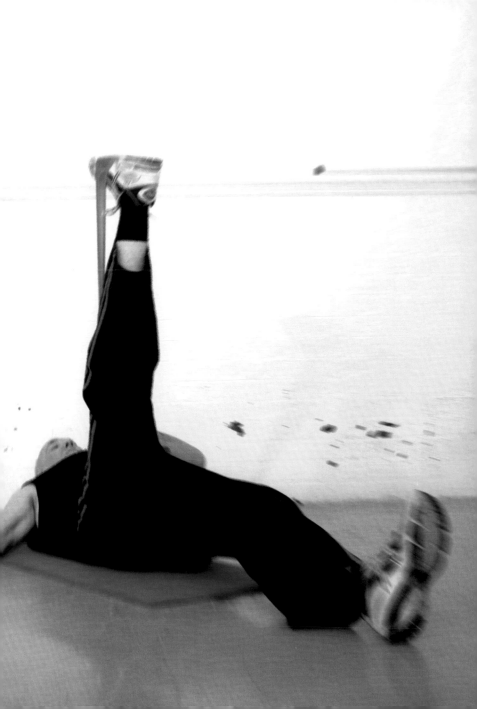

35. Working-Out with Bands and Tubes

Using only bands and tubes can still give you a good resistance workout; the important factor is that the rubber is tensed throughout the exercise, it is important to always take up any slack. By the same token always bear in mind that even top quality rubber products of this nature are only sound stretched to up to three times their original length. If this limit is exceeded it will not perform properly, leading to distortion or breakage.

Select the correct strength of rubber product by testing yourself with ten repetitions of an exercise you intend to be part of your workout; you may need two different bands of varied strengths:

One for large muscle group exercises e.g. chest press, lat pull downs and squats

One for smaller muscle group exercises e.g. bicep curls, tricep press.

For Safety's Sake

Remember the rubber has a limited life expectancy estimated at about 20,000 stretches – you don't have to count; you will be able to detect when your equipment is "going home." A rough guide would be about two years life expectancy.

If the rubber is exposed to sunlight, extreme cold or hot temperatures, salt or chlorinated water, its life span will be even shorter.

Don't wear your sparklers when training – sharp edges from rings or fingernails can cause tears and weaken them. Always check your bands for damage; if a tear is detected you may as well discard them as they could snap on you without warning.

Do not try knotting two lengths of tubing together to form a longer unit – this is a recipe for disaster.

The downside of training with bands is they have some limitations with regard to working all muscle groups efficiently without some form of contrivance. Even this drawback can be reduced by introducing some additional products to secure or anchor the tubing or band to facilitate exercises.

The upside is that both bands and tubes are easy to store, are portable (can be taken on holiday) and are relatively inexpensive, none of which can be said of weights.

Bands are usually about £3 each, but a roll of tubing, which can be cut with scissors to form individual bands of the required length, costs around £30, which can work out cheaper if bought by a group of friends or family.

Testimony

With his 60th birthday looming, Harry Newson (a lifelong friend) was disturbed to see his weight had ballooned to over 16 stone. In order to combat his growing proportions and to improve his health generally, he and his wife, Trisha, set out on a course of moderate exercise and sensible home-cooked food. As they travel widely and needed something they could take with them, they started training with Tricord bands, which they bought in John Lewis for £24.99, which included three different strength bands and padded handles and a 40 minute instructional DVD showing 12 exercises. Harry had, he estimated, not exercised for 25 years (probably even more in my estimation) apart from playing golf, during which he would always take a buggy.

Only a couple of months into his new regime, he reduced his weight to 14 stone 10lb: not a drastic reduction but nevertheless sensible. The major benefit was how much better and fitter the pair of them felt, even if Harry is going to have to splash out for a new wardrobe.

If you haven't got a DVD player, or got hold of a suitable book on the subject – here are some exercises you can make a start with. The DVD and book that often accompanies a set of bands will include compound exercises, which involve working two muscle groups at once e.g. shoulder press and calf raise, but my workout is aimed at people who are just trying out this mode of exercising, and for that reason I have deliberately kept it simple and assumed the user has nothing to hand except for the tube. Using immovable objects, such as stair hand-rails can give a useful base for such exercises as 'lat pull-downs' and 'seated rows'; if you decide at a more advanced stage of your training to incorporate this idea, always ensure the object is immoveable (steer clear of household pipes and cables). Most of the companies that sell tubes, sell stabilising equipment advertised as *safety door anchors* to affix your tubes to doors or stair-posts.

Tubes Workout

Warm-up: 5 minutes of aerobic exercise (jog on spot, skip, static cycle or shadow box).

Punching incorporating band

Mobilise joints (as before)

Short stretch (as before)

Suitable for all levels;

Repetitions for different levels:

Level 1: 2 sets of 10 repetitions

Level 2: 2 sets of 12 repetitions

Level 3: 3 sets of 12 repetitions

Level 4: 4-6 sets of 12 repetitions

Where it indicates a single arm working below (exercises 3, 10, 11, 12), the number of repetitions refers to actual number on that side, therefore total repetitions for one completed set will be double the above.

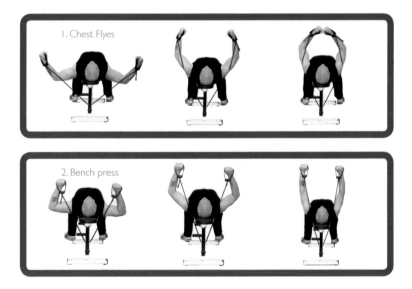

1. Chest Flyes

2. Bench press

3. Single arm rows

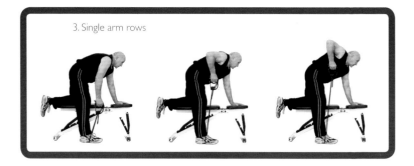

4. Seated rows

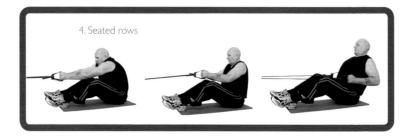

5. Shoulder press (shoulders)

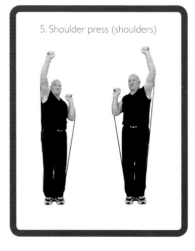

6. Lateral raise (shoulders)

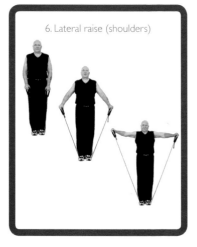

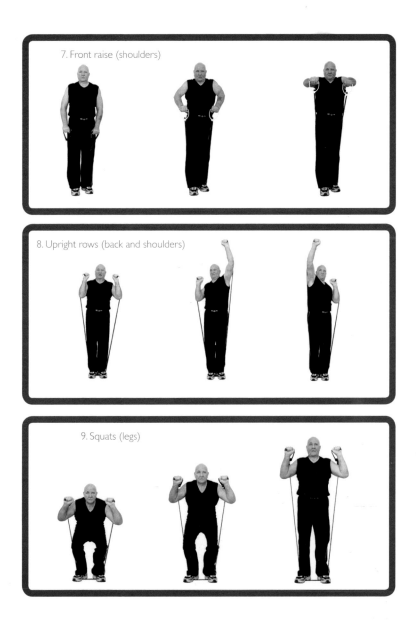

7. Front raise (shoulders)

8. Upright rows (back and shoulders)

9. Squats (legs)

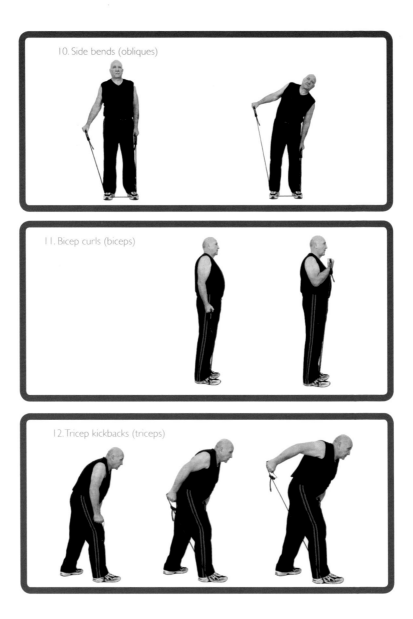

10. Side bends (obliques)

11. Bicep curls (biceps)

12. Tricep kickbacks (triceps)

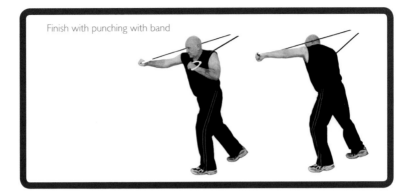

Finish with punching with band

■ 5 minutes aerobic exercise (same as warm-up).

■ Cool-down stretch, flexibility and mobilisation.

This workout includes no abdominal work and I would advocate inserting some crunches, planks, reverse curls into the workout in the interests of giving it balance.

■ Level 4 trainers could also include press-ups.

36. Golf

The very mention of the name can send certain individuals into an anti-golf rant, or can mean an arcane world in which people derive enjoyment from striking a small ball with expensive and cumbersome equipment. I was in the 'indifferent' school, pretty much as I still remain with regard to angling and horse-racing; I can understand why people enjoy them, but it is not for me. A relatively short while ago, my friends, aided and abetted by my wife, dragged me into the sport which, like skiing, I wish I'd started earlier, but was hardly in a position to do so. I have to admit to having become a total convert; even when my friends Dave Clow and John Hayes and I have played the most dreadful round of golf known to mankind we still agree – it beats working. Few can argue that it is an healthy outdoor pursuit, involving much walking, interrupted by light physical activity.

The Benefits

Tones leg muscles.

Improves cardiovascular endurance.

Lowers cholesterol.

Increases metabolism, thereby burning more calories.

Taking Steps

Medical experts have given a guideline of 10,000 steps a day as the target distance to achieve and maintain a reasonable level of fitness. Clip your pedometer on one day when you set off for eighteen holes of golf and you will generally find you will, according to the size of the course, be doing in excess of 12,000 steps, more if you include walking to and fro looking for lost balls.

Golf and the mature person's blood pressure

The benefit I have not included is blood pressure. I cannot say, with my hand on my heart, that golf will reduce your blood pressure; this depends upon the individual's attitude to a series of frustrating setbacks: losing golf balls in streams and ponds, missing the ball with an 'air-shot', going 'out of bounds' with drives, duffing, slicing, hooking, shanking and many, many more pitfalls that await the fledgling golfer. I have to say that if you are ultra-competitive, not prepared to laugh at yourself and expect quick results, then if you are over 50 years of age golf will not be good for your blood pressure. That said, if you have played any sort of hand-eye coordinative sport in the past (like tennis, football, cricket, netball, or hockey) and have a reasonable degree of patience, golf is a great new adventure for the mature person. You stroll through woodland and meadow, enjoying the beauty of your surroundings, in pleasant company of like-minded individuals (just so long as they're not thrashing you), while feeling the benefit of healthy exercise.

When you start

Get some lessons from a professional. I feel anybody over 50 starting golf will benefit vastly by getting lessons from a professional. Lessons start from around £15 a session at my modest club, but if you sign up for a course they will work out cheaper and you are going to need a few. This is where you can drop the hint that when your birthday comes around, golf lessons might be nice.

Equipment, Courses and Clubs

You do not have to take out a second mortgage to acquire golf clubs, but simply buy what you can afford. Some courses will hire out clubs, but I have seen starter kits, complete with bag, for under £100. Again, the local press usually has some bargains in second-hand kit, as somebody trades up to more sophisticated gear, or gives it up as a bad job.

If you take lessons you do not need any clubs, as the pro will provide them, and also be in a position to advise you when you are ready to purchase your own.

Once you have your clubs it is well worth investing in a comfortable pair of golf shoes; many clubs allow flat-soled trainers, and while I have no problem with this, some members get a little snooty. Check out the club regulations before you consider joining to ascertain whether or not the rules are too stringent for you. I feel the 'downmarket' clubs are a good way of attracting new people, especially kids and older folk who have retired with only a state pension to rely on, and those from the less well-off areas of society. It is nice to see older people going round the course with their grandchildren.

If you do not want to join a club there are numerous *pay and play* courses, many run by local councils and invariably in good condition. *Pitch and putt* courses are usually cheap and cheerful and great fun.

Once you feel ready to venture forth don't fret if you have nobody to partner you. Golf is the most sociable of sports, and if two people arrive at the first tee at the same time it is usually the case they will go round together. Many people are without a regular partner, but it is likely the pro knows who most of them are, especially if they have been to him for lessons, and will usually find lone players somebody to pair up with them. Don't worry if they are vastly better and more experienced than you. It's like learning to drive: most sensible people are patient with a learner. We all had to start somewhere.

Never Mind The Weather

Waterproofs are an essential piece of kit. Get a jacket and over-trousers that can be rolled up and stuffed in a pocket of your golf bag. As with walking, take a hat with a peak; it will shield you from the sun and when the rains come protect those who wear spectacles from near blindness. Pack a bottle of water in the summer; if you are walking a few miles you do not want to dehydrate.

Buggies, Backpackers and Trolleys

A friend of mine informed me he played golf to 'get some exercise' but admitted he always hires a buggy. Pure common sense dictates that a buggy removes the major ingredient of exercise. Only take the buggy if you have a disability or the course declares it mandatory. If you find the bag is too heavy for you to carry, then hire or buy a trolley, or you can usually hire a trolley from the club. Electric trolleys are, like the buggy, designed to conserve energy rather than expend it. Why would a perfectly fit person need an electric trolley? I wouldn't expect my wife to lug a full set of clubs around but she gets a good enough workout hauling it along on her wheel-along trolley.

Tote that bag

If you want to get some positive physical exercise while playing then carry your bag, which allows legwork and resistance for improved fitness.

Don't carry your bag over your shoulder for too great a time, instead look for a bag with straps like a rucksack, which comes with a spring-out stand when you put it down. The weight of the bag, once adjusted to give equal weight on either side of the lower back, pulls the shoulders back and helps to maintain good posture while walking; good form while carrying can help strengthen the muscles of the back and shoulders and the extra weight helps to tone the leg muscles.

I recently spoke to a disconsolate octogenarian who bemoaned the fact his arthritis had stopped him carrying his bag any longer and he had been forced to resort, reluctantly, to a pull-along trolley.

Home in on the Range

If you are unsure if you will like golf or not why not find out by hitting some balls on the driving range. Most clubs will charge £2-3 for a bucket/basket and usually offer a '6 for the price of 5' offer. It is a great stress relief to just launch a few dozen balls into the ether, whether they fly straight or not. The beauty of the range is that most of them are floodlit and stay open until late.

Get Fitter, Get Better

As with most sports the fitter you are the better you are likely to perform, and, contrary to what many may think, golf is no exception. You are not only going to be walking for 2-5 miles every time you play (and so you need a reasonable level of endurance) but you are going to require strength to get distance from your strokes. Technique is paramount, but swinging a club about a hundred times in a game (fewer on a good day, more on a bad one) is going to make demands of your body strength, so it helps to be in shape.

Since people learned that Tiger Woods and many of the current leading golfers train with weights, aspiring young golfers are doing the same, but it is never too late for golfers of any age to give themselves a little more of an edge. I see guys with what looks like a beach ball under their jumper, probably good players, restricted to a half swing because their gut does not allow more movement.

You can find specific golf fitness programmes but I feel a combination of all-body weight training and regular stretching to improve flexibility, will help immensely.

A Word of Warning

Remember golf is a rotation sport and will make demands of the upper body; if you have had problems with your back or shoulders in the past, speak to your doctor before taking it up, or speak to a fitness professional about strengthening the specific area likely to be troublesome.

High compressive loads are placed on the spine during a golf swing, and if you are aware that you suffer from osteoporosis it would be inadvisable to start swinging a club vigorously; medical advice must be taken in this case.

Specific Strength and Flexibility

Apart from the regular strength training you will find in this book try these exercises and stretches which target the muscles used in golf:

Strength

- Semi rotations with hand weight or medicine ball

- Never full rotation, which can cause spinal injuries

- Wrist rolls – over and under

- Dumbbell side bends

Flexibility

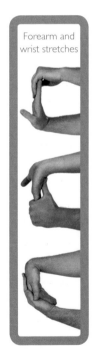

Forearm and wrist stretches

Forearm stretch

Semi-rotations using long golf club

Side bends with golf club

Wrist rolls – clockwise and anti-clockwise

Head turn – both sides slow

Chin drop (slow)

Sky gazer (head drops backward) slow

Shoulder rolls – to and fro

Ankle rolls

A Personal View

    I did not think for one moment I would ever play golf, let alone enjoy doing so, but I have to say I enjoy it as much as all the other sports I have participated in, even if I am as mediocre in ability as I was at most of them. My aim is nothing greater than being competent. If I ever do better than that I shall feel elated. I will never fully learn or understand all the rules, but then even the pros often ask for a ruling, so what chance do I have?

    I can in all honesty only advocate sports or exercises I have tried myself at some stage, and for mature people golf is probably the one I would most heartily endorse, with regard to its mildly physical exercise and its social aspect.

    Golf was once considered only available to the more privileged or wealthy sections of community, but it is now within the scope of anybody who fancies trying it; its recent popularity lies in the fact that, unlike most outdoor sports, it can be played in all weathers, and it encourages a high level of sportsmanship, to the point that the onus is on the individual to play to a faultless degree of honesty – I never found that in football or cricket, as much as I love them both.

    You have nothing to lose but a few hundred golf balls and, possibly, your sanity.

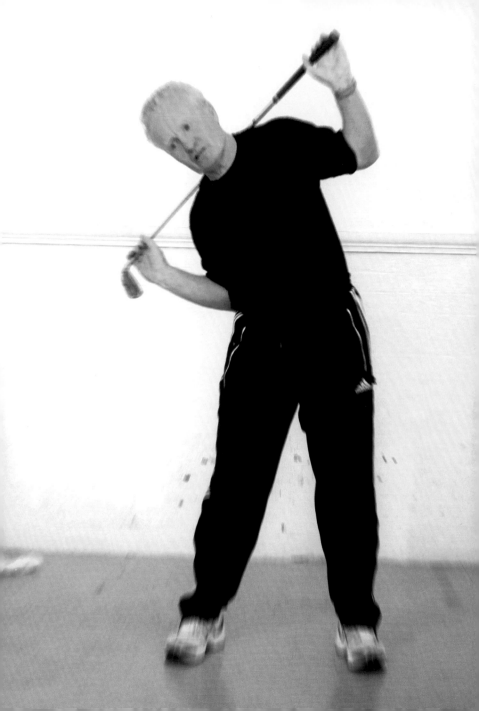

37. Tennis

Tennis, like most racquet sports, requires some degree of residual fitness when you start, as you will be called upon to make sharp movements at regular intervals. Tennis fitness is fairly specific. You do not need to be a superbly conditioned athlete to enjoy this terrific sport – I have seen obese people turn in a decent game of tennis – but a reasonable fitness level will be advantageous. It should, according to how regularly and how intensely you play, improve your fitness immensely.

If you feel you would like to get into tennis but are unsure of how to start, look up your local club and see if they run coaching sessions. Observe a session first and judge whether or not you are likely to enjoy it (both the coaching and the atmosphere).

Coaching is to be encouraged, although many people are self-taught or learn from manuals – there are hundreds to choose from. However, a coach will encourage good technique by using drills and basic learning techniques. A coach will also tell you what you should look for when buying a tennis racquet and a coach will discourage bad habits and enforce the good ones, giving you confidence in your game.

The obvious drawback is the weather; it is soul destroying to arrive at the courts just as the heavens open and play becomes impossible. Try to find a club with all-weather courts, as grass courts demand higher technique and become unplayable following prolonged rainfall.

As far as fitness is concerned, there is a gulf between singles and doubles tennis. In singles you are using frequent bursts of high energy, albeit interspersed with rest periods. In doubles you are more likely to be only half as much employed, according to the fitness and ability of your partner. I would endorse both singles and doubles play, but people following levels 1 and 2 will be best suited to doubles tennis until they attain level 3 fitness. Even if the weather is not warm, I would still advocate carrying a drink in your bag to ensure you are hydrated, especially in hotter climates, should you play while abroad. Make sure you have a cap with a brim for those rare occasions when the sun bursts through to blind you, and wear proper footwear with a decent amount of tread on the sole for grip.

John Wahlers is a friend and a former football team mate of mine, for a good many years. I feel his experience of taking up tennis in his fifties is a good testimony to the enjoyment of the sport. He retired from playing football and became a referee, but was looking for something other than simply refereeing at weekends.

John writes;

"How can I keep fit whilst I am unable to officiate at soccer matches?" This was my dilemma in my early fifties, which was brought about by a short term inability to give commitment and availability to refereeing, due to family illness.

The answer was tennis, which enabled me to remain very active and also join my wife, who had been a member of the Marconi Tennis Club in Chelmsford for several years.

Tennis is an ideal sport, offering different levels of playing standard and involvement. There are also social elements, on and off court. Choose a club carefully, to suit your playing ability and potential. Look closely at the facilities and the friendliness of the members. Tennis can be very competitive on the one level, which suited me fine, but it can also provide friendly sociable activity.

A good way to start is to join a club's group coaching sessions for members and non-members alike. This will help you gauge how friendly and helpful the coaches and the members are. It also allows the coaches to assess your ability and potential whilst improving your game.

My involvement in tennis grew. On court, it was league matches and club tournaments; off court, it was as a committee member and organising a men's singles

ladder. More recently my wife and I have taken over
the running of a tennis holiday in Portugal for
club members and other friends we have made through
tennis.
When circumstances allowed me to get back into
football refereeing, after much soul-searching, I
had to say no.
I decided I had put enough back into football, a
sport which had been so good to me over many years.
It was time to move on. Although I sometimes wonder,
I have no regrets.

John Wahlers, January 2006

Warm-up, Stretching and Mobility

A quick jog or running in place for a few minutes, followed by a relaxed knock up will serve as a warm-up; space and facilities can be limited in respect to warming up and warming-down.

Take a minute or two to go through the "one minute (short) stretch".

Tennis players must mobilise the joints, especially in cooler weather:

Head turns to loosen neck muscles

Arm rotations to loosen shoulder muscles

Hip circling

Knee hugs to loosen gluteals

Wrist rolls

Ankle rolls

A warm-down stretch, if there is no provision to lay down should be as the short stretch but with individual stretches extended to 20-30 seconds each.

Fit for the Game

Just as in most sports, serious-minded participants can improve their tennis with a good overall, well-balanced fitness programme. Weight training will improve strength, circuit training and running/jogging will improve endurance, and skipping, in particular, will improve upper/lower body co-ordination as well as stamina like few other exercises can.

> *"Revise your expectations of who can learn from whom - there's nobody out there who can't teach you an important lesson about something."*
>
> From Roddick A., Agassi A., and Gilbert B, "I've Got Your Back: Coaching Top Performers from Center Court to the Corner Office" (2004) Portfolio.
> Andy Roddick's and Andre Agassi's tennis coach. Brad Gilbert

38. Injury and Illness

Once you start training you can get yourself into great shape, but you also run the slight risk of injury, mild or otherwise.

As soon as you feel any pain or marked discomfort – stop training! Rest the painful area immediately, which will reduce circulation and thereby allow the tissue to begin the repairing process.

If your injury turns out to be of a long-term nature, it does not necessarily mean you cannot train at all. Do what you can, within the bounds of common sense and comfort. Leg injuries, according to severity, do not mean you can't still train your upper body, just as something like a sprained wrist or elbow ligament problems will not prevent leg training.

Do not put off getting a chronic problem examined professionally. If you get no satisfaction with the National Health Service (some do, some don't) see a private specialist, get an estimate for a single appointment first. By doing this, you should: speed up the treatment, find out the root cause of your problem and how to prevent re-occurrence.

There are books available to teach you how to do your own massage, which is not as tricky as it may at first appear, and which can, with a little patience, prove very beneficial (see "Massage and Self-Massage" page 282).

Make sure you are warm enough when you train outdoors, cold muscle fibres do not respond well to being extended. On a hot summer day, cover your head to protect against sunstroke or train at a cooler time of day.

If you turn up late at the gym don't save time by skipping your warm-up, joint mobilising or stretching, skip an exercise instead.

When buying equipment, as long as you can afford to, go to a store that gives expert advice be it on weights, footwear, cycles or machines.

When buying sports shoes, try to do so later in the day when your feet will be a little larger, by as much as 5%. Tight-fitting shoes can lead to all sorts of foot problems. Blisters are a common problem with people who have recently taken up walking or running. To prevent them re-occurring, smear the soles of your feet with a coating of Vaseline. Treat blisters by dressing them with a 'blister pack', available from pharmacists, and keep them clean to avoid infection if the skin is broken.

Illness

Inevitably, there will be times when you will fall prey to the odd cold. The general rule of thumb regarding training is: if it's from the neck up (sniffles but not a head injury!) train lightly; if it's from the neck down (aching limbs, coughing, wheezing, feeling lethargic) do not train at all.

When returning to training after illness or injury, ease your way back into your regime; you cannot catch up on lost time by overworking, so don't try to.

If friends, family or training partners tell you that you look unwell or off-colour, take notice and proceed carefully; you might just be coming down with something. Curiously enough, nobody wants to share your illness, and gyms are a great place to catch something contagious or infectious, so be considerate.

First Aid

Familiarise yourself with the basic procedure to follow if a training partner incurs an injury. The very minimum you should know and remember is "RICE".

R = rest—stop training now!

I = ice—get some ice, very cold water or freeze-spray applied to the injury as soon as possible, and try to keep it on for 20 minutes every hour. With ice, wrap in a towel first, to prevent ice burn.

C = compression—apply a firm bandage or strapping to prevent painful movement and limit swelling.

E = elevation—raise the injured limb to allow blood to flow back to the heart.

RICE is the most basic first aid advice, but is quite easy to remember and put into effect. Obviously if the injured person is in agony or has suffered a major trauma, do not do anything other than call for an ambulance as quickly as possible, then making them as comfortable as you can while they wait for professional medical assistance.

A one-day first-aid course is relatively inexpensive and many local councils have them running continuously. Attending such a course counts not only for your own welfare in a crisis, but for friends, family and more usually, total strangers. I signed up for a course many years ago after a youngish man from an opposing football team collapsed with a heart attack in the dressing room, directly after the game and, out of the many people at the ground only the referee knew what action to take.

Train Sensibly

Don't take unnecessary risks like carrying on when in pain, going out running on icy pavements or foggy evenings.

Never train vigorously in extremes of temperature, especially heat; try to train at the cooler part of the day and ensure you keep your fluid content up.

Try to always get a decent night's sleep, but if you have had a rough, sleepless night, don't train too hard the next day.

Calf problems

Calf pain is a common problem with runners and can occur for a number of reasons, some avoidable, and some which need professional advice to appertain why they re-occur. The avoidable is usually poor technique or inadequate footwear. Those comfy old trainers may need closer inspection, especially if they have a heel tab that is causing friction, or if the sole is worn and the insole completely knackered. Go to a specialist running shop for a shoe specific to your needs (see running shoe advice on page 107).

If you feel the onset of a nagging pain in the calf while out running/jogging, then slow to a stop and walk to your destination – you cannot 'run it off'. Continuing to run can aggravate the injury considerably. On reaching home, or the changing room, get some ice on it as quickly as possible (see home ice massage kit below). After this carry on the R.I.C.E. procedure and start stretching as soon as the pain subsides, in order to retain flexibility. If walking is difficult try inserting a ready-made heel support of sorbothane or supple sponge rubber.

In addition to the calf stretches shown on page 54, there are other specific calf stretches you can supplement your recovery with:

The 'Doorstep stretch'

Supporting your upper body, allow your heels to overhang the edge of a step or stair. Lean forward and allow your heels to drop as low as they can. Hold this for 10-15 seconds. Then perform the same stretch with your heels turned out to give a pigeon-toed effect, and again but with the heels closer together in a 'ten to two' Charlie Chaplin stance (for more mature readers).

Tiptoe walking

Simply walk around, bare foot, on the tips of your toes, until your calf muscles ache.

Exercise band stretch

Take an exercise band and loop it around your bare feet while seated. While pulling on the band, push your toes forward against the resistance. This can be done with a leather or fabric belt if it is long enough to do the job.

Cramp

Another calf problem is that of cramping. The usual course of action is to lay on the ground while somebody holds your heel and forces the sole and toes of your foot downward. Untrained muscles run the highest risk of falling victim to cramp. This technique will most likely relieve the spasm, but if it continues a vigorous massage should be tried next. I trained football teams long enough to appreciate the efficacy of both methods. If you have nobody around to manipulate your foot, press your toe against a hard surface (e.g. a wall or a tree) and lean forward to stretch the calf muscle. If this fails, self-massage comes next. You will need to rub the affected area vigorously, while gritting your teeth in all likelihood.

The causes of cramp are considered to be a deficit of fluid, salt, calcium or magnesium. My personal experience was that habitual cramp sufferers prevented its onset by eating a packet of crisps an hour or two before a match, purely for the salt content. Others swear by eating a banana or a bowl of cereal and milk; if you are a regular cramp sufferer you can experiment to find your cure, but frequent attacks should be discussed with your G.P. in case there is a serious underlying problem involving blood circulation.

Shin Splints

With this injury, pain is felt at the front of the lower leg, along the shinbone. It can often start out as a nagging ache but gradually increase, with activity, into a quite painful and debilitating condition. It is usually caused by landing during running/jogging, football or other activities involving bounding, on hard or uneven surfaces. Amateur footballers often sustain this injury at the beginning of the season, when their new boots come in contact with hard grounds, as do novice runners setting out on hard pavements. Technique and footwear should both be carefully scrutinised to prevent re-occurrence once recovery is complete and training is resumed.

Self-help involves using ice as soon as possible (see home ice massage kit below). As soon as pain allows start stretching by pulling your toes towards you, preferably against a resistance for more effect; sit down and insert your toes under a heavy bench, then extend your legs fully until you feel the affect of the action on the injury site. Alternatively get a friend, preferably one of slight build, to stand on your toes as you recline, or press against your feet with their hands.

> **Tip**
>
> Both Achilles problems and shin splints can also be caused by increasing the intensity of training too quickly. There is a need to allow time for the body to adapt to increased demands by gradual increments; try not to step up the level of your training too rapidly.

Sprains

1. Ankle

There are, commonly, two types of ankle sprain, damaging either the lateral (outside area), or the medial (inside area).

1. An *inversion* injury is likely to injure ligaments on the outside (lateral) side of the ankle. This is the more common injury because there is greater movement in inversion.

2. An *eversion* injury is likely to injure ligaments on the inside (medial) side of the ankle. This is less common because there is less movement in eversion.

Sprains are generally caused by the ankle 'going over' on an uneven surface, a stumble when moving quickly, or, in my case, missing the edge of a kerb in bad light.

At first you may think, (as I did), "I've only twisted my ankle, it might be all right." When you arrive home the pain has often grown, and so has your ankle – usually to twice the normal size.

Your foot starts to feel hot, and the dull ache becomes sickeningly painful and tender to the touch, and any movement is jarring – yes, it's not just a twist, it's a sprain.

Plunge your foot into a bowl, or better still, a 'decorator's bucket', a rectangular one, that will allow all the foot to fit in fully extended, fill with cold water and empty the contents of your ice tray into the water, while gritting your teeth. Failing this, wrap a packet of frozen peas around the affected side and secure with a tea towel or a long sock, and rest your injured leg over the arm of the sofa. From here on follow R.I.C.E. procedure, but it is always worth getting a doctor to look at the injury, who may suspect a fracture and send you for an X-Ray to make sure.

Once the swelling and pain subside, usually about one to two weeks, start to exercise your ankle by rotating in both directions, and with up and down movement of the foot, to improve mobility and flexibility. Roll a tennis ball around with your bare foot to improve strength and control in the ankle.

2. Wrist Sprain

The wrist is another joint susceptible to sprains, usually incurred by a heavy fall or being wrenched during exercise or working. As before plunge the affected limb into a bowl or bucket of cold water with a generous helping of ice cubes. As with the ankle it is worth getting a doctor's opinion in case it is not just a sprain but a fracture.

Once the pain and swelling allow get the joint moving again and try some wrist strengthening exercises using a small dumbbell or a soup can.

Upward roll

Hold the weight over the edge of a bench or table, palm facing upward. Slowly bring the hand up towards you, knuckles facing towards you. Try to do 3 sets of 10 repetitions

Downward roll

Hold the weight over the edge of the surface with palm facing down. Slowly bring the weight upward as far as you can, with back of the hand facing you. Try to do 3 sets of 10 repetitions.

Invest in a squash ball or one of those squishy sponge balls made for this purpose and carry in the car to use when sitting in traffic, or in your pocket to squeeze while waiting for bus, tube or train, or while viewing something mind-numbing on television or reading the newspaper - double-tasking that works for everybody.

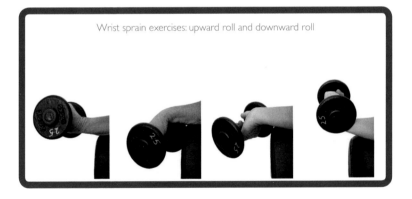

Wrist sprain exercises: upward roll and downward roll

Massage and Self Massage

Massage is an ancient healing art and can often achieve outstanding results where other healing has failed. It relaxes tired bodies and eases stiff muscles and joints. A session with a professional masseur/masseuse is wonderful, but if you need regular massage it can become expensive. Home massage is an alternative.

In the list of useful literature I have included "Sports and Remedial Massage", by Mel Cash and "The Complete Guide to Massage" by Susan Mumford, both of which have a chapter on self massage. The second book is good for total beginners who want to learn how to massage or self-massage.

Massage oil can be bought ready-made, but it is equally effective and much cheaper to make your own. Use almond oil or rape seed oil as the carrier oil (the bulk liquid), although baby oil or olive oil will do, and then add the essence of your choice, be it lavender, camomile, peppermint or any from the enormous range available. My personal choice is lavender, not only because a knowledgeable osteopath advised it, but because it smells so good. If you have aching muscles lemongrass would be a particularly good choice.

The mix – get a plastic bottle that will not leak; you don't want everything in your bag to reek of essence. Fill the bottle up to the shoulders (about 80% full), then add 2-3 drips of essence to a small bottle, or 7-8 drips into a half-litre bottle. Shake vigorously. A half-litre bottle of rape seed oil from the supermarket costs a little over a pound. A bottle of essence from Sainsbury's, Tesco or Body Shop, Holland and Barrett or any health store, costs around £3, and lasts for ages. For around £4 you have a long-term supply of massage oil, all you have to do now is rub it in; a massage book will tell you the exact technique, but if you rub towards the heart until the skin reddens, that will be a good start; apply the oil to warm hands, then to the area requiring massage. Never apply oil directly to the body.

Ice Massage

You can use this handy little device anywhere, but I have found it is extremely useful on strains in the calf muscle.

Take a Styrofoam cup, (one of those that break into thousands of little white balls that get everywhere when crushed) and fill to the brim with cold water.

Place container in your freezer.

At the first onset of a mildly strained muscle take the container and cut around the brim with a sharp knife to remove the top half of an inch.

Massage the hard protruding ice around the injured site until the ice softens and becomes unusable. Concentrate solely on the exact site of the injury, don't widen the area that you ice.

Time over small areas should be about 5-10 minutes.

Replace cup in freezer.

Repeat every time you require it, until it is too small to be practical. For this reason keep two or three on the go at one time.

If the strain is particularly painful use R.I.C.E. procedure instead.

(my thanks to Savash Mustafa, an osteopath, for medical advice in this section)

Back Pain and Prevention

While exercise can provide an extremely good chance of preventing back pain, the hope of reversing acute back pain through exercise is not supported by clinical evidence. While exercise can improve the overall health of back pain sufferers, it is unlikely that exercise can, at this stage, help improve back problems.

There are three main categories which relate to physical activity and back problems:

1. For those who are currently well and disease free, they can benefit by using physical activity for maintaining and improving their fitness, especially incorporating exercises targeted at strengthening the back and the core muscles (e.g. rowing, weight-training, core training).

2. For those who already suffer from back problems on occasion, but are not chronic, it makes sense they select exercise that is not going to aggravate the back. Medical consultation would be advisable in this case.

3. For those with established back pain, who will need exercise that does not involve the afflicted area, but will improve their general health.

The majority of back pain problems are not due to bad luck, but to a history of poor posture. Work-related back pain is the largest workplace-related injury issue, and is responsible for an estimated 25% of workplace health expenses (Straker, 2000). As the computer age advances apace, 'white-collar' back and neck pain keeps stride with it due to long hours hunched over the keyboard, despite recommendations to regularly 'get up and walk around'. I would advise adding 'stretch as you walk' to this advice.

When bending forward from the waist, always try to support the body; forward flexion of the upper body without support is a recipe for disaster.

Other possible causes and considerations are:

- Weak abdominal muscles, which offer no support to the back to keep it erect, so the best exercise for your back happens at the front; try to build a steely corset for your back with abdominal and core exercises.

- Lack of flexibility can also be responsible for back pain, where mobility and suppleness of the legs and backs has been neglected. For this reason alone it is important to improve your flexibility with regular stretching and mobilising.

- Life for the back can be improved if people are carrying less weight around the middle, making it easier for the back to straighten once it doesn't have to hoist the additional weight of something equivalent to a holiday-packed suitcase.

- Help yourself by sleeping on a firm mattress, sleeping on your side, and sitting up in bed by pushing up sideways with your arms as opposed to sitting up by bending forward from the waist.

- The message to those fortunate enough not to suffer from back pain is – don't take it for granted. Exercise now can prevent crippling pain further down the road, so start thinking about a strength training plan that will keep you pain free and mobile.

Osteopath Savash Mustafa states:

"Those with established back pain will need exercise that does not aggravate their back problems. In addition they will require professional medical advice.

Many back problems are greatly helped by specific rehabilitation exercises, again professional help is needed."

Getting to the Foot of it

The older we get the more likely we are to have foot problems. This kind of problem can obviously impair physical functioning and balance problems, which may increase the likelihood of a fall.

The skin on the feet of older people becomes thinner and drier, making it less resilient. Ligaments also change with age, affecting the structure and function of the foot. An increase in weight can also result in spreading the foot, resulting in a flat-foot condition.

All older people should have their feet checked out regularly, especially if their feet have been troublesome or painful; medical intervention can successfully manage many of these problems.

Chronic conditions, such as flat feet can be assisted by the use of arch supports or orthotic innersoles to get the wearer back on the move. Orthotics are being used more and more these days (I wear them myself for running to combat plantar fasciitis). Orthotics can be obtained after referral to a National Health Physiotherapist, or you could have them tailor-made for anywhere from £150 to £300.

The bottom line is that under no circumstances should you endure painful feet; see your doctor, he may feel you need to see a foot specialist.

(See 'Choosing Footwear' in "Running/Jogging" page 107 & "Walking" pages 90-91)

> *"It is health that is the real wealth and not pieces of gold and silver"*
>
> Mahatma Gandhi

> *"Growing old is like being increasingly penalized for a crime you haven't committed"*
>
> Anthony Powell – Temporary Kings 1973

39. The 'Subjects'

The following people were foolhardy enough to see if a training plan devised for them would help them achieve improved fitness and weight loss.

Joyce

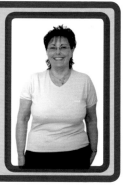

Aged 61, housewife and babysitter to two lively granddaughters (aged 3 and 7). Joyce gradually eased herself into getting fitter, joining a gym being a major first for her, but she is slowly going from strength to strength, amazing her friends and family.

Sally

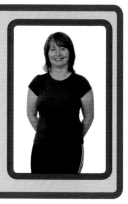

Aged 50, combining part-time work as a management consultant with being the perfect housewife to husband Rodney, and mum to Alex 21, and Beth 20. Sally has trained particularly hard and achieved a well-merited result; just watching her work out is enough to make many feel weary, what is heartening is how much she has actually enjoyed it.

Doug

Aged 50, a busy company director, married with grown-up children and a two-year old at home. Due to a heavy workload Doug admits he has been "shirking" his training, particularly his cardiovascular content, although he does ride his bike for transport whenever possible. He has managed only one session of training a week (sometimes none at all) with my colleague Wayne Rowlands, a martial arts instructor; I feel this is the

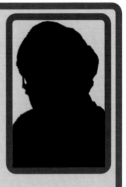

only way he could have lowered his pulse and made emphatic strength gains. On seeing his results, particularly the weight gain and body fat increase, he has vowed to embark on doing at least a two-day plan of rowing and circuit training, in addition to his martial arts session. We shall see…

Alex

Aged 57, Alex works as a councillor to people with learning difficulties and, part time, as a Martial Arts Instructor specialising in grappling. Living with partner Lyn. Known to one and all as "Big Al", for reasons he was not altogether happy about, especially when he realised around December 2004 he was hitting the scales at 22 stone. He decided to take positive action and, as his results show, he is currently just over 16 stone, looking

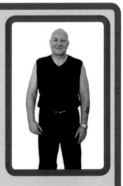

lean and still a bit mean. He has earned even more of our respect for his metamorphosis. He is still Big Al to all, but the reference is now to his heart and his persona, rather than his girth.

The Fitness Tests

The fitness tests carried out can quite easily be done at home.

Blood Pressure (normal blood pressure 100-140 systolic/ 60-90 diastolic)

Your G.P. can take this for you with unerring accuracy when you visit the surgery, but a home blood pressure is reasonably accurate enough to help you keep an eye out for hypertension. Your blood pressure should be taken when you are at rest.

The monitor used in all the tests was an Omron Upper Arm Blood Pressure Monitor, costing around £67. A large cuff for those with a broad upper arm is available from A&D for around £17. The monitor also gives a pulse reading, but I used the 'pulse at the wrist and stopwatch' technique, which I favour. For the benefit of anybody who has not taken their own pulse, simply place your 'watch hand', (you will need a watch with a second hand facility), across your other wrist, with the middle three fingers across the radial artery, just below the base of the thumb. If you have difficulty getting a 'beat', try placing your fingers at the side of your neck (the carotid artery). Count how many beats you feel in 60 seconds for the most accurate reading, or ten seconds multiplied by six for an approximation.

Peak Flow

To gain an accurate idea of lung function I used a Mini-Wright Peak Flow Meter, which retail at around £11. Operation is simple, you just take a good blow into the tube and the gauge records your reading.

Body Fat

The body fat tests were conducted using an Omron Body Fat Monitor (hand held variety) which retails at around £50. I checked the results using 'Slimguide Calipers'. These threatening-looking but, nonetheless harmless, gauges, cost around £18, and are accurate, but need to be taken, preferably, by somebody using correct technique. They are impractical to use on oneself, unlike the Omron Monitor, which is extremely user-friendly.

The meter also records Body Mass Index (BMI), but if you do not have a monitor you can calculate it for yourself using the following method – reach for the calculator first, and be prepared to 'go metric'.

You will need to:

Divide your weight, in kilograms by your height, in metres squared (I said you'd need the calculator).

So – if you weigh 10 stone, that will be 63.5 kilos

You are 5' 6", that will be 1.67 metres

Which, when squared = 2.79

Divide 63.5 by 2.79 = 22.76

Which will be your BMI, (give or take a 0.01 here or there).

There are charts which will tell you what your BMI should be, but I just feel they don't take body or 'soma' types (see chapter on Body Types pages 32-34) into consideration. Keep an eye on your BMI when you exercise and try to keep it under 27, if you can. If it is over 30, try to bring it down.

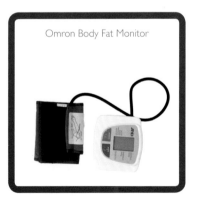

Omron Body Fat Monitor

Bike Tests

The bike tests were taken all on the same machine, a Keiser Static Cycle. All four subjects rode for five minutes at the same pace.

Press-ups

All four people did the maximum amount of press-ups they could manage, before collapsing in a heap.

Curl-ups

These are not sit-ups! All four subjects simply laid on a floor mat with bent knees, hands resting on thighs; they then curled forward until their fingertips reached their knees. The numbers recorded were the actual maximum they could achieve.

Plank Time

Time spent resting on elbows and knees (the kind version) for as long as was sustainable (see abdominal training, 'the plank', levels 1 & 2 pages 63-64).

I tried in the main not to be too fussy about the tests. These people were not about to be launched into space or ascend Everest, they just wanted to get a little fitter, so we had a few laughs when we carried them out, as I hope you may if you decide to try a little 'home-testing'.

Alex's Fitness Assessment

Motivation

In December of 2004 I went on holiday over the Christmas and New Year period. I had booked a two-centre holiday, one week on a cruise ship and a week in a hotel. On Christmas Day we visited the island of Madeira, where I had my photograph taken and was horrified to see from it just how much weight I had put on. On arriving back at the ship I went off to the gym and weighed myself. Well, there was no avoiding it, no excuses that I could use – I was 22 stone 4lb! My chest measurement was over 50 inches, and so was my waist!

The Plan

My plan was that I would eat healthily for the next two weeks; the food was very good and prepared to a high standard, and I had sufficient knowledge to devise a specific diet plan for myself. I did not cut down; in fact I ate more than I would have normally. I also did a lot of walking in the second week around the holiday resort we were based in, which I believe also had a bearing on my weight loss of almost a stone (21st 2lb) in two weeks. With this success I decided to keep to the healthy eating programme.

Further Motivation

A week after I arrived back from holiday my doctor called me in for a hypertension screen, as I was over 55 years of age. So the next shock in store for me was to discover I had high blood pressure and that my doctor would be prescribing medication for this. I was not very happy about this, and began to look into ways I could help myself. I trawled the internet and found something called the DASH eating plan, which stands for the Dietary Approaches to Stop Hypertension eating plan. This was not a weight-reducing diet; it was about simply eating healthily, and I embarked on this plan. I soon noticed I was losing more weight – so no more sausage and chips for me (I had got into the habit of eating 'convenience' food at least three times a week).

The Fitness Plan

To keep the weight loss going I decided to walk to and fro to my workplace. I was making good progress, having now reduced my weight by almost three stone, now down to 19st 2lb, but my fitness was showing only minor improvement. I was still having problems climbing the three flights of stairs to my office and I could only do a pitiful 5 push-ups and 10 curl-ups. My plan had to have a method to get me fit and feel better in myself.

The Damascus Moment

Like Paul on the road to Damascus, my moment of insight came when I picked up Ian Oliver's book "*Boxing Fitness*".

Ian and I were both instructors at The Academy (a boxing gym), but I had never discussed my weight or fitness with him. I had looked at a great deal of fitness books over the years and found most to be quite boring. After reading the first five or so pages I bought the book and, once I started reading it I had finished it from cover to cover in a day or two. I started doing 'The Solo Training Workout', once a week initially, moving on to twice weekly. I was so impressed with this I asked Ian to devise a specific weight-training plan for me, which he did. I have continued with this plan and the solo workout for several months. This has motivated me to join a large gym, so that I could continue with my workouts in the hours that The Academy was closed.

One Year On

This has been a journey of discovery for me; the holiday photograph and the hypertension results had prompted me to change my lifestyle radically. No longer the couch potato, but somebody who got off his rather large rear end and did something about it. My current weight loss is around 6 stone and has been a steady reduction over the last 12 months. My fitness level has gone up so much I can do now do 50 push-ups and 40 sit-ups, and I now run to work daily! My blood pressure has come down to within the normal range and I will be asking my doctor to review my medication. I do not have so many headaches and generally feel so much better in myself.

This fitness programme has had such a positive effect on all aspects of my life; I believe it is something I will continue with from here on in. The daily food diary that Ian suggested I keep has helped me to stay on track, and to stay focused on my eating habits.

Now a word about skipping, which I saw was included in the workout. I have never skipped and was of the 'don't skip, won't skip' school. Incredibly, I now carry a skipping rope and a timer with me all of the time, so I can fill in any spare time with two or three minutes of skipping.

The downside of all this is that I have had to buy new clothes, clean out my wardrobe, throwing out the 'big stuff', much to my partner's joy.

I would like to thank Ian Oliver for one, writing his book "Boxing Fitness" and two, giving me the help and encouragement to go on. Thanks also to the staff of Bob Breen's Academy, London, for all their support.

At the time of writing my weight is now 16st 6lb.

Doug's Fitness Assessment

Given that his fitness tests didn't come out too well, I didn't ask Doug to make an assessment, as the others have done. He simply admitted his work has kept him away from the gym, apart from an hour-long martial arts session, when he can manage it.

Having studied his results, with some horror, regarding his weight and body fat, he realises he must get down to some serious time management in order to get some cardiovascular exercise content into his week. What his test fails to show is the enormous strides he had made in the previous year, he would admit his physical condition was quite poor when he first started training, but improved considerably.

As stated in the earlier chapter, 'Muscles have Memories', Doug is going to have to give his muscles a few clues to remind them what he wants out of them.

Joyce's Fitness Assessment

Starting My Programme

It only took about an hour to do the exercise programme every other day but I found it difficult to find time to fit it in.

Warming up was boring, I tried jumping on a trampoline, running up and down stairs – it was all so boring, I didn't want to start.

Doing a food diary was repetitive – how many different things can you eat?

What I Enjoyed

I enjoyed doing the weights and stretches, I only found the warm up boring, but I knew I had to persevere. I then decided to join a gym – now, that's a real first for me, I still can't believe I've done it. I liked the idea of the swimming pool, as I only ever swim on holiday.

What I Disliked or Most Found Most Difficult

I was restricted during the week to Wednesday and Thursday, as the classes I liked were on those days. Some family members were negative at times, with a "you won't stick to this" attitude. In addition, family commitments make it difficult at times.

The Cost

The cost of joining the gym is £36 per month, plus some clothing, swimsuit, jogging trousers etc. The cost alone will urge me to go, as the more classes I take – the cheaper they become. Just call me Mrs Scrooge.

The Benefits/Unexpected Benefits

I actually feel fitter; have slightly more 'puff' than before. I've also lost some weight, not much, but now I'm more determined to keep my weight going in a downward direction. I've got into the habit of swimming more, and am doing low impact aerobics and Pilates.

I tried several classes to start with, but now do aerobics, Pilates and Aqua Tone. There is no point in doing what I don't enjoy.

I also use the Treadmill and Cross-Trainer (though I don't really like this one very much).

I now realise that you have to be fit to be old, so exercise has to be part of my new life, nothing too fanatical, but just enjoyable.

Diet

I did not really change my diet whilst following the exercise programme as I already have a restricted diet. I should not eat wheat or dairy as it really does not agree with me. However I did find keeping a food diary very useful because it showed me that I did eat wheat and dairy, and also that I probably drink too much!

A food diary also has a strange psychological effect on you. Firstly, you think, "I had better not eat that as I will have to write it down", even if no-one else is going to see your diary. Secondly, your mind can convince you that you haven't eaten chips every day, but your diary is evidence that, in fact, you have.

So although I did not change my diet I was probably more aware of what I was eating. It did not stop me enjoying my food or a glass of wine, but it did help to prevent excess.

Sally's Fitness Assessment

Starting My Programme

Starting something is always the hardest part and my fitness programme was no different. It was not the exercise that was hard but organising myself to find the best times to train on a regular basis.

I decided to do the weight training element at home and the boxing workout at the gym before I started work. I set Mondays and Wednesdays for my boxing circuit and Tuesdays and Sundays for the weights. If I missed a day I could train on the other days and retain my rest days. I did my weights programme while watching television.

I found out very quickly that I needed new training shoes. My shoes were worn and as soon as I looked in the mirror I could see that they offered no support and definitely had no bounce left in them.

For myself, and any other woman, a good sports bra is a must – just try skipping without one! I need not say more.

I would also recommend that when you initially do your training programme, if you need reading glasses – take them with you. I made the mistake of not taking mine before I was familiar with the programme. I then mistook some 1's for 2's and found myself doing 2 minutes of fast skipping instead of one! Take my word for it, it makes a huge difference. I thought Ian was particularly mean until I realised my mistake.

What I Enjoyed

In the first two weeks I enjoyed the fact that, when I went to sleep, I was sleeping soundly until the morning, and that a feeling of calm was creeping over me. After a few weeks I could work hard all the way through each set of my programme. After a few more weeks, particularly when running or skipping, I felt the "ping" and "bounce"

I remember from my younger days was returning. That was a lovely feeling.

I also enjoyed the gradual re-emergence of a waist. After the first six weeks I had lost two inches from my bust, two inches from my waist and three inches from each thigh!

What I Found Difficult

That moment before you start your workout; the "chicken out" moment. Thoughts such as "I could just not do this and go and have a nice cup of coffee instead," arose. But once I had pulled myself together and started training, when my blood was pumping a bit harder, it then became very enjoyable. It is the getting the bum off the seat that is the hardest part. Once the decision is made, the training is relatively easy.

Costs

Warning! There are hidden costs with Ian's programme, which surprised me. I had to buy new clothes in smaller sizes as my other clothes began to hang on me. Be warned!

The best bit was trying on a size 12 that turned out to be too big. I had to go for a size 10 for the first time since I was 28! Admittedly it was a Marks and Spencer size 10, and not a Top Shop size 10, but I knew that even if I had more training to do, I was on the right path.

Benefits

I am feeling much fitter and more confident in myself and in my fitness. I feel altogether more feminine and less sluggish. I feel more physically and mentally vibrant.

It was funny, I was really impressed with my results, but Ian wasn't at all surprised – "it's a structured programme, it will work." I expect Ian is used to seeing results, however, in future, Ian, could you just say "Wow!"?

Unexpected Benefits

Aches and pains that I had in my shoulder from an old accident, and a general weakness in my knees when going up stairs, completely disappeared. I sleep better and have become extremely calm. Another surprise was how my flexibility improved; I am not sure if was the result of the exercise, the stretching, or a combination of the two, but it was very welcome.

I discovered how much I love boxing training, especially hitting the punch bag. I am now keen to learn some new techniques and add some kickboxing. It is not hard to train if you are doing something you enjoy.

It is hard to start to get fit but once you see the benefits it is a pleasure to continue. Although, in life, responsibilities and events can sometimes make it difficult to train, the benefits are too great and too joyous to ignore.

> *"Success is a journey, not a destination"*
>
> Bruce Lee

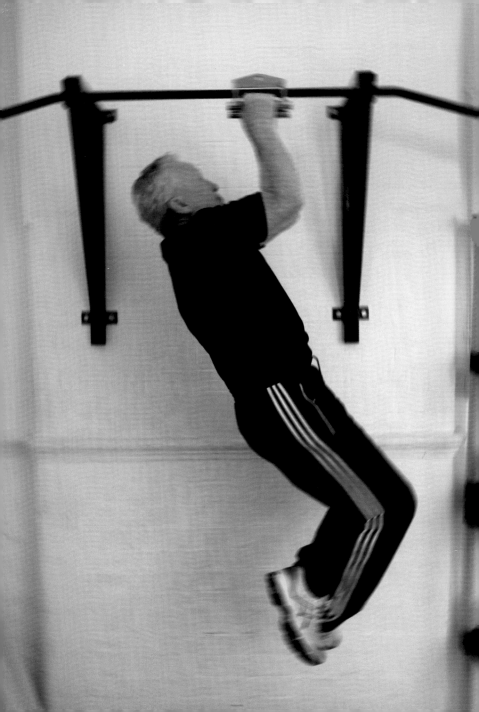

40. Handy Kit

These items are all mentioned elsewhere in this book. Here is a little more detail about them.

Pedometer

These useful little items have been about for years, but have lately, given the earth-shattering news that walking is actually good for your health, undergone a renaissance. They used to record the mere detail of how many steps you have taken, but you can now get pedometers that will relate amount of calories burned, speed in mph or kph, steps per minute, as well as providing time, date, stopwatch, radio, panic alarm and ones that talk to you (complete with funny looks from fellow-passengers on public transport), a wireless variety for greater accuracy (estimated at 98%) and some come complete with a compatible wristwatch. Some are interactive and can have their information downloaded onto your computer, others are built into watches.

Some need to be clipped to the belt, others sense movement even if in your bag. I have seen them as low-priced as £2.99 for the low-end model, £24.99 for a sophisticated model and up to £100 for high-end, it all depends on the level of gadgetry. Whichever way you look at it, if you only need to know how many steps you have taken and how far you have travelled then a basic model should suffice.

While the model you buy may not have NASA-type accuracy it will at least be consistent for your individual performance, showing you if you have walked further or faster.

Timer

If you are going to do any form of training where you need to work for a set time, then an inexpensive digital timer is a boon.

Just set it, start it and forget all about it until it bleeps. I picked one up from Sainsbury's kitchen accessory department for £2.24 and to my delight, it is idiot proof and comes with a strong clip and a magnetic plate.

Press-up Stands

These stands take pressure off the wrists, allow a greater range of downward movement and at £3.99 are a steal.

Second Hand Fitness - the unwanted and unloved treasures of the small-ads column.

Other people's rejects and junk can be the answer to your fitness problem. Why splash out a small fortune on weights when somebody is selling "York weightlifting bench" for £14! Old weights weigh the same as new ones and if you want to get fit you won't be bothered about the aesthetic appearance of your weights and bench. Even if plates have traces of rust a quick coat of Hammerite paint will sort that out. Likewise, a full set of golf clubs, replete with trolley and golf balls must be worth the £40 being asked, to the complete beginner thinking of taking up the game.

Ebay is another source of bargain fitness equipment, but if you want to have a good look at the kit first you know the people who advertise in the local paper will be close enough for a visit, and won't charge postage.

Packing for the Gym

Not as extensive as packing for a holiday, but imagine your annoyance when you discover you haven't packed a towel, drying yourself on a t-shirt isn't quite the same. If you are not the owner of a razor-sharp memory or a born organiser, make a quick list, especially if you are a newcomer to gyms. When buying a sports bag consider how much kit you intend to tote around; will you be taking your own yoga mat? Some items well worth including, in addition to the obvious showering requirements, are:

Flip-flops

Avoid foot infections, particularly verrucas, they are harder to get rid of than a tattoo.

Plastic bag

To keep your wet stuff away from items you want to keep dry, and avoid getting that mouldy odour in your bag.

Water bottle

Stay hydrated, get a large one, fill from the tap and sip as you train. A sports bottle costs around £3-4 and are designed to be easy to grip.

Skipping rope

If you intend to skip at the gym, take your own rope as theirs may all be in use, or too long/short for you (see Skipping – Choosing a rope page 160-162).

Warm-up gear

If the gym has a tendency to be on the cool side, or somebody has been over-zealous with the air conditioning, throw in a warm sweatshirt, which you can peel off once you are warm. If it is really cold, pack a woolly hat and track trousers. Don't start exercising cold muscles when it is avoidable.

Petroleum jelly (Vaseline)

If you are wearing anything new or have some sensitive areas of skin, apply some Vaseline to appropriate areas to prevent chafing and soreness.

Small hand towel

To mop your fevered brow and any equipment on which you may have left evidence of your efforts.

Also useful:

- Small packet of plasters

- Small (nail) scissors

- Packet of tissues and medi-wipes.

- Safety pins

- Pen and small writing pad for note-taking, memos etc.

Books - Further Reading

Anderson B, 'Stretching' (2000) Pelham Practical Sports

Balk M. and Shields A, 'The Art of Running: With The Alexander Technique' (2000) Ashgrove Publishing

Barough N, 'Walking for Fitness' (2004) Dorling Kindersley

Bean A, 'Food for Fitness: Nutrition Plan, Eating Plan, Recipes' (2002) A & C Black

Bean A, 'The Complete Guide to Strength Training' (2005) A & C Black

Dr. Bird W, 'Walking for Health and Happiness' (2002) Reader's Digest Association

Brand Miller J, 'The New Glucose Revolution' (3rd Edition) (2003) Hodder Mobius

Cash M, 'Sports and Remedial Massage Therapy' (1996) Ebury Press

Clark N, 'Nancy Clark's Sports Nutrition Guidebook' (1989) Human Kinetics Europe Ltd.

Delavier F, 'Strength Training Anatomy' (2005) Human Kinetics Europe Ltd.

Dixon J, 'Swimming Coaching' (1996) Crowood Press Ltd.

Edwards S, 'The Heart Rate Monitor Book' (1993) Leisure Systems International

Fiatarone Singh M.A. "Exercise, Nutrition and the Older Woman: Wellness for Women over Fifty" (2000) CRC Press Inc. US.

Galloway J, 'Running: Getting Started' (2005) Meyer & Meyer Books

Grisogono V, 'Sports Injuries' (1994) Crossing Press.

Guzman R. J, 'Swimming Drills for Every Stroke' (1998) Human Kinetics Europe Ltd.

King M, 'Pilates, the Complete Body System' (2003) Mitchell Beazley

Kowalchic C, 'The Complete Book of Running for Women' (2000) Simon & Schuster Inc.

Lee B, 'Jump Rope Training' (2003) Human Kinetics Europe Ltd.

McCord G, 'Golf for Dummies' (2006) Hungry Minds Inc.

Moran G. T. and Pearl B, 'Getting Stronger: Weight training for men and women' (2001) Shelter Publications Inc.

Mumford S, 'The New Complete Guide to Massage' (2006) Hamlyn

Norris C, 'The Complete Guide to Stretching' (2004) A & C Black

Schoo A. "Optimizing Exercise and Physical Activity in Older People" (2003) Butterworth-Heinemann Ltd

Sharkey B, 'Fitness and Health' (2001) Human Kinetics Europe Ltd.

Slater N, 'Real Fast Food' (1996) Overlook Press

The St John Ambulance Association and British Red Cross 'First Aid Manual' (2002) Dorling Kindersley

Walker M. and Wright N, 'Women's Golf: The Ultimate Instruction Guide' (2002) Hamlyn

Westlake L, 'Strong to the Core: Get on the ball for a strong, lean physique' (2003) Aurum Press

It stands to reason that not all these books will suit everybody, I have simply picked out what are user-friendly guides for specific activities. The ones I have found to be the most loaned out from my collection are:

'The Complete Guide to Strength Training', by Anita Bean. This well-written book is so simple to follow and helpful for people of all ages.

'Nancy Clark's 'Nutrition Guidebook'—thorough in every detail from a true expert in this field, although the Anita Bean nutrition book runs it pretty close.

'Sports Injuries' by Vivian Grisogono—a practical self-help guide, and I just happen to know a lot of people who pick up niggling injuries.

'Strength Training Anatomy', by Frederick Delavier. There is now a women's version of this book, which gives superbly illustrated and well-documented weight-training exercise in every precise detail. Everybody I have loaned it to has gone on to buy his or her own copy; it is almost indispensable to anybody who enjoys weight training.

I never loan Brian Sharkey's 'Fitness and Health' to anybody, for fear of losing it; I regard it with awe as the best and most accessible book on every aspect of physical health. I cannot recommend it highly enough.

Most libraries' health and fitness sections have a wealth of books which provide rich resources – for free – so make the most of it. I cannot believe how few people ignore this wonderful facility when trying to improve their fitness or sporting ability.

Health and Fitness Glossary

These terms may appear obvious to many, but to be absolutely sure I feel I should define the following terms in the context of this book:

Aerobic exercise - Exercise 'with oxygen', literally. Builds cardiovascular improvement. An example of aerobic exercise is jogging during which you should be capable of conversation with a partner.

Alexander Technique - A technique for positioning and moving the body that is believed to reduce tension.

Anaerobic exercise - Exercise 'without oxygen', literally. Strenuous exercise that uses oxygen faster than the blood can supply it. An example is sprinting, as this form of exercise can only be sustained for short periods.

BMI - Body mass index, calculated by taking body weight in kilograms by the square of the height in metres.

BPM - Beats per minute, another way of saying 'heart rate'.

Calisthenics - Gymnastic exercises designed to develop muscular tone and promote physical well-being.

Calorie - Unit of energy, where one calorie is the amount of energy needed to raise the temperature of 1 gram of water by 1 degree centigrade.

Carcinogenic - Containing an agent capable of causing cancer.

Chronic - Term describing a disorder or set of symptoms that has persisted for a long time. A chronic illness is where such an illness continues with little change in symptoms with the passage of time.

Core - As in 'Core Training'. The deep abdominal and back muscles that give support to the spine and lower back.

DOMS (also known as DMS) - Delayed onset muscle soreness. Usually occurs at its worst two days after training. Often due to excessive training and lack of rest and recovery. Sufferers should examine their training programme and technique to prevent reoccurrence.

Exercise - Physical activity set out to achieve a positive result.

Fitness - How well you perform physical activity.

Health - Wellbeing relating to your physical and mental condition.

Jogger's nipple - Soreness caused by chafing/rubbing of garment against the nipple of men or women, usually while jogging or similar activity.

Lactic Acid - A syrupy, water-soluble liquid, produced in muscles as a result of anaerobic glucose metabolism.

Ligament - A band of strong, fibrous tissue found in joints of the body, binding bones together while allowing limited movement but prevent excessive movement.

MHR - Maximum heart rate, roughly calculated for men as 220 - your age and women as 230 - your (honest) age (e.g 50 year-old woman = MHR of 180 bpm).

Morbidity - The state or condition of being diseased in medical statistics.

Obesity - A condition in which excess fat has accumulated in the body. A person 20% above the recommended weight for his or her height is considered obese rather than overweight.

Osteopenia - Low bone mass.

Osteoporosis - Loss of bone tissue, causing the bone to become brittle and increased risk of fracture.

Physical activity - Movement caused by muscular action that requires energy to perform.

Pilates - A method of physical and mental exercise involving stretches and breathing that focus on strengthening the abdominal core. Etymology: Joseph Pilates, designer of the system.

Repetition - One performance of a particular exercise, commonly used in resistance work. A 'ten rep max' refers to a set of exercises where the first repetition is easy but by the tenth it becomes challenging.

Repetitions - Each completed movement of a particular exercise is described as a 'repetition', (even if it is not repeating anything, it is possible, but unusual except in bodybuilding, to perform 1 repetition).

Set - Term used in resistance training to describe a number of repetitions. A general workout for a beginner would be a "3 set, 10 rep" schedule.

Somatotype - The structure or build of a person, especially to the extent to which it exhibits the characteristics of an *ectomorph*, an *endomorph*, or a *mesomorph*.

Tai chi - A Chinese system of physical exercises designed especially for self-defence and meditation.

Tear drop bag - A pear-shaped, hanging punch bag.

Tendon - A band of fibrous, flexible tissue which attaches muscle to bone or muscle to muscle.

Yoga - A Hindu discipline aimed at training the consciousness for a state of perfect spiritual insight and tranquillity. Also a system of exercises practised as part of this discipline to promote control of the body and mind.

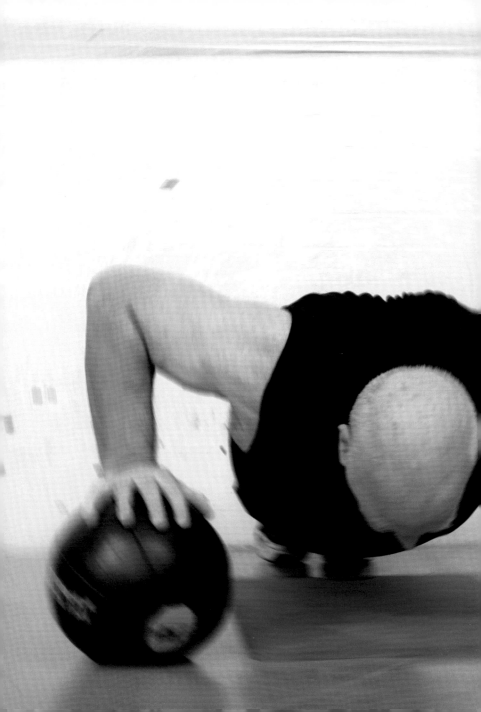

Stockists

Asics

UK Address: | Asics UK Ltd.

Europa Boulevard,

Westbrook

Warrington

Cheshire, WA5 5YS

Telephone Number: | 44-1925-241041

Fax Number: | 44-1925-414894

Email Address: | info@asics.co.uk

Website Address: | www.asics.co.uk

US Address: | Asics America Corporation

16275 Laguna Canyon Road

Irvine, CA 92618

Telephone Number: | (800) 678-9436

Email Address: | consumer@asicamerica.com

Website Address: | www.asicsamerica.com

Concept2, Inc.

Address UK: | Concept2 UK Ltd.

Vermont House, unit 5

Nottingham South & Wilfred Ind. Estate

Ruddington Lane, Wilford,

Nottingham, NG11 7HQ

Telephone number:	0115-945-5522
Fax number:	0115-945-5533
Email:	info@concept2.co.uk
Website:	www.concept2.co.uk
Address US:	Concept2, Inc.
	105 Industrial Park Drive,
	Morrisville, VT 05661, USA
Telephone number:	800-245-5676/ 802-888-7971
Fax number:	802-888-4791
Email:	rowing@concept2.com

Coolmax

Address:	INVISTA Building
	4123 East 37th Street
	North Wichita, KS 67220
Telephone number:	1-302-774-1178
Email address:	invistainfo@invista.com
Website address:	www.coolmax.invista.com

Dans-ez®

Address:	Dans-ez International Ltd
	7 Blenheim Close
	Pysons Road Ind. Estate
	Broadstairs,
	Kent, CT10 2YF
Telephone Number:	+44 (0) 1843 866 300

Fax Number:	+44 (0) 1843 860 880
Email Address:	sales@dans-ez.co.uk
Website Address:	www.dans-ez.com

Dynaband®

Address:	PO Box 1195
	Naphill, High Wycombe
	HP14 4WQ
Telephone number:	0870-850-4133
Website:	www.dynaband.co.uk

"Dynaband® are available from John Lewis stores and most sports shops."

Everlast Boxing

Address:	Everlast Boxing
	14711 West 112th Street
	Lenexa, KS 66215
Telephone Number:	1-800-777-0313
Fax Number:	1-913-492-7546
Email Address:	info@everlastboxing.com
Website Address:	www.everlastboxing.com

Gold's Gym

Address:	The Sports Nutrition Company Ltd.
	Unit B, Easting Business Centre
	Easting Close
	Worthing, BN14 8HQ

Telephone Number:	01903 820 808
Fax Number:	01903 820 234
Email Address:	info@sncdirect.co.uk

Keiser Corporation

Address:	2470 South Cherry Avenue,
	Fresno, California 93706-5004 USA
Telephone number:	559-256-800/ 800-888-7009
Fax number:	559-256-8100
Website adress:	www.keiser.com

Life Fitness UK Ltd.

Address:	Queen Adelaide
	Ely, Cambridgeshire, CB7 4UB
Telephone number:	01353-666017
Fax number:	01353-666018
Website address:	www.lifefitness.com

Nautilus

International Address:	Nautilus International SA
	Rue Jean Prouve 6
	1762 Givisiez
	Switzerland
Telephone Number:	+41 (0) 26460 7777
Faz Number:	+41 (0) 26460 7770
US Telephone Nunmer:	(800) 782-4799
US email address:	email@nautilus.com

Website Address:	www.nautilus.com

Reebok Fitness Equipment

UK Address:	DFDS house
	Maidstone Road
	Milton Keynes, MK10 0AJ
Telephone number:	01908 512244
Website address:	www.rbk.com
US Adress:	ICON Health and Fitness
	Reebok Consumer Service Department
	1500 South 100 West
	Logan, T 84321
Telephone number:	1-888-308-9621
Website address:	www.reebokhomefitness.co.uk